Dr. Karine Aloyan

An Infectious Disease Physician on the Backstage during this Pandemic

Dr. Karine Aloyan

An Infectious Disease Physician on the Backstage during this Pandemic

JustFiction Edition

Imprint

Any brand names and product names mentioned in this book are subject to trademark, brand or patent protection and are trademarks or registered trademarks of their respective holders. The use of brand names, product names, common names, trade names, product descriptions etc. even without a particular marking in this work is in no way to be construed to mean that such names may be regarded as unrestricted in respect of trademark and brand protection legislation and could thus be used by anyone.

Cover image: www.ingimage.com

Publisher:
JustFiction! Edition
is a trademark of
Dodo Books Indian Ocean Ltd. and OmniScriptum S.R.L publishing group

120 High Road, East Finchley, London, N2 9ED, United Kingdom
Str. Armeneasca 28/1, office 1, Chisinau MD-2012, Republic of Moldova, Europe
Managing Directors: Ieva Konstantinova, Victoria Ursu
info@omniscriptum.com

Printed at: see last page
ISBN: 978-620-3-57549-1

Table of Contents

Abbreviations

BMI	Body Mass Index
COVID-19	Coronavirus (COronaVIrus) Disease-2019
HIV	Human Immunodeficiency Virus
H1N1	Hemagglutinin Type 1 and Neuraminidase Type 1, a strain of influenza virus causing swine flu
MERS-CoV	Middle East Respiratory Syndrome – Coronavirus
RN exam	more precisely NCLEX-RN exam - the National Council Licensure Examination – Registered Nurses, is a national exam that all nursing students must pass to become licensed registered nurses in the United States
RT-PCR	Reverse Transcription - Polymerase Chain Reaction; one of the most accurate diagnostic methods to diagnose various diseases, including COVID-19
SARS-CoV, SARS-CoV1	Severe Acute Respiratory Syndrome - Coronavirus 1
USMLE	United States Medical License Exam
WHO	World Health Organization
2019-nCoV, SARS-CoV-2	2019-novel Coronavirus later named Severe Acute Respiratory Syndrome – Coronavirus 2

<h1 align="center">Medical terms used in the book</h1>

Asymptomatic – with neither signs and symptoms; nor pathological changes. Just specific analysis for a concrete disease may diagnose the disease. Compare with "**Pre-symptomatic**" – no signs and symptoms yet.

Causative agent – an alive organism, substance, or phenomenon that causes disease.

Cholecystitis – Inflammation of the gallbladder.

Coinfection – concurrent infection with two different causative agents.

Coronary arteriography – the most accurate method to define the extent and severity of blocked vessels supplying the heart.

Dementia - loss of memory, language, problem-solving and other abilities that are severe enough to interfere with daily life.

Diverticulitis – inflammation or infection of small bulging pouches in the digestive tract.

Emerging disease – a disease whose incidence (the number of new cases) in humans has increased in the past 2 decades or threaten to increase soon.

Exanthem – skin rash. Compare with "**enanthem**", rash on mucous membranes, for example, in the oral cavity or on the conjunctiva.

Exogenous and endogenous – outside or inside of the body, respectively.

Facultative pathogenic microorganism – a microorganism that usually resides in the host organism and causes diseases when contributing conditions happen. "Pathogenic" means able to cause disease.

Hemoptysis – coughing up blood.

Human Herpesvirus 6 – a representative from Herpes family not yet fully investigated. It causes the disease named sudden exanthem (exanthema subitum) observed almost always in little kids.

Incidence - number of new cases of a disease, condition, symptom, death, or injury that develop within a defined timeframe, such as a month, a year. Compare with "**prevalence**" - the number of new and old cases of a disease minus death cases in a particular population at a given time.

Myocardial infarction – blockage of bloodstream to the heart muscle followed by its death.

Oxygen saturation – the amount of oxygen bound to blood cells expressed in percentage.

Pathogenesis – the chains of events inside the host organism leading to disease development.

Petechiae - pinpoint, round spots due to bleeding into the skin do not turn pale after pressure applied.

Prenatal or postnatal – before or after childbirth, correspondingly (can refer not only to the mother or newborn, - but also to the father).

Primary prevention – intervention to prevent the disease or bad condition to happen, examples, vaccinations, smoking cessation, development of healthy habits.

Postpartum – after delivery (refers to mother and a newborn).

Reinfection – infection with the same agent after recovery.

Resection - the surgical removal of part of an organ or structure.

Reservoir – an organism in which an infectious agent (bacterium, virus, or other) able to cause disease in other species lives and multiplies typically without damaging the host organism itself.

Resistance gene – a gene determining partial or no effect of an antibiotic or disinfecting substance.

Secondary prevention – measures to diagnose the disease early-stage once it has already developed, to treat properly, and to prevent complications.

Site of entry – tissue or organ via which the causative agent enters a host organism.

Sporadic – infrequent or irregular occurrence of a disease. Compare with "**outbreak**", a sudden increase of cases is excessive from expected.

Subclinical – without signs (objective presentation of the disease) or symptoms (subjective presentation, i.e., complaints) but with pathological changes that can be established via usual laboratory or instrumental assessment, such as complete blood count, liver markers, CT scan, or ultrasound.

Superinfection – infection superimposed by the inner or external agent before recovery.

Thromboembolic complication - formation in a blood vessel of a clot (thrombus) that breaks loose and is carried by the bloodstream (embolus) to plug another vessel.

Zoonotic disease – a disease that can be transmitted from animals to humans.

January 2020

Missed wake-up call

"Doctor, what do you think about this novel coronavirus?", "Ensure us that it is just a local infection", "Do you think it is going to be more serious than swine flu?", "Will it spread all over the world?", "The scientists will find the treatment and vaccine soon, won't they?" … Hundreds of similar questions are being addressed to me by my students, friends, relatives, and colleagues all over the world. They still trust my opinion even though they know that I am not currently in practice.

I am an infectious disease physician with ten-year practical and eight-year academic experience. It has been two years since I moved to the United States from Armenia. My medical carrier was quite successful for a small, developing country. Nevertheless, for the last few years, I started seeing my professional future abroad when I realized my potential cannot be fully unlocked in Armenia. After weighing all the pros and cons and struggling with two steps of the United States Medical License Exam (USMLE), I came to Los Angeles as a tourist for another USMLE. With limited finances and having no one in the medical field to direct me, I was about to go back home as soon as I would receive the exam results. My cousin Emmy who lives in New York with her family; invited me to join them. She moved to the United States many years ago, made an amazing carrier, and created a wonderful family. Since my childhood, she was one of the few people inspiring me, however, we have not seen each other for about eighteen years. Despite such a long time passed, I felt at home. Emmy helped me as only the eldest sister could do. She supported me in every little or great problem one can face in a foreign country. While I was on pins and needles waiting for medical residency interviews that every physician should pass for the license to practice medicine in the United States, crucial changes in my personal life appeared on the horizon. A man who I saw several times in California visited me in New York and proposed. Victor is a son of my parent's friends who came to the United States twenty years ago. Our last meeting with them was at New Year in Yerevan when I was a cute little girl and had obliged to stand on a chair singing and reciting poems for our guests. Who might imagine then that the young handsome guy I was so shy of would become my husband? Despite the short period of our acquaintance as mature people, I did not doubt my choice. I finally found a real soul-mate next to who I felt as reached home after a long and tiresome journey. The only tough decision concerned the time of marriage: to go back and return in six months or to overstay and continue building our relationship. Both I and Victor imagine the family as a precious tree to be grown from a small seed, to be watered on time, to be cared for thoroughly, and to be protected from excessive sun and storms. As our relationship was in the stage of sprouting, we did not want to risk it with time and distance. The person who always obeyed laws and rules, who would "never take two toothpicks or napkins instead of one" stated by my friends, decided to risk and to overstay. While I and my fiancé were changing attorneys one after one, arranging my documents for legal status another deadline to apply for medical residency had passed. We often sacrifice one thing for another, a more treasured thing. This time it was my carrier for my love and family. And if I had to choose again, I would do the same taking both happy and horrible consequences on me.

So, in January 2020 I am a beloved wife, a new mom, a homemaker, and seemingly a useless physician. My son Eddy is two months old. His mild but prolonged jaundice has just resolved, he grows up so fast still being a terrible sleeper. Victor puts a lot of effort into his job trying to meet all the needs of our growing family. I set many stores by his attempts, however, being physically alone, sleepless, and unable to leave Eddy without crying for more than five minutes is backbreaking. My parents-in-law live nearby, they visit us almost every day and are incredibly supportive, even so, Eddy does not stay with them longer than allowing me to take a shower fast and to do a few house chores. He sleeps requiring my presence, so between "sleep when your baby sleeps" and "keep studying" I choose the latter one. Postgraduate online programs, news, and articles from the world's best medical journals, podcasts, webinars start to replace the absence of jobs, friends, and leisure.

I have never stopped being a physician at least in my mind and heart. I dreamed to become a physician since my early childhood, weathered numerous storms such as family resistance against my choice and incredible competition, admitted and graduated with honor a quite corrupted medical university without any assistance, gained employment at the best clinics of Armenia, tasted the bitterness of reaching high levels in the desired profession without proper wages. But I never quit medicine! Being a physician is not wearing a white gown that I may take off when I finish my job. It is rather a way of life, a way of thinking, a big part of me! In public, I often unwillingly scan people's general constitution, gait, behavior, mood, and perceive their visible or barely noticeable medical problems trying to help them at least in my mind. I am eager to study and enrich my medical knowledge every day. Victor recognizes my shining eyes when I reveal interesting medical news or the answers to my questions. He even stated once "it looks like being on a date with the beloved one". Now, when the novel coronavirus appeared endangering the world, I receive dozens of messages daily. It is time to share my mastery as much as possible. Informed, means armed, at least partially.

-   Doctor Karine, what is the coronavirus? It is the same "cold virus", isn't it?

- Coronaviruses is a virus family causing an illness named "common cold" that is more prevalent in cold seasons, hence in the nonmedical language it is often explained as "just catching a cold due to bad weather or low temperatures" or "being not dressed for the weather". However, coronavirus infections – more than just the common cold. We have known at least two highly pathogenic coronaviruses: severe acute respiratory syndrome coronavirus (SARS-CoV) and Middle East respiratory syndrome coronavirus (MERS-CoV). They emerged from animal reservoirs, a phenomenon that happens with other microbes, as well. Even though these two coronaviruses appeared with alarming morbidity and mortality, they did not spread across the globe. It is still unclear how the current coronavirus will behave, but as a professional in infectious diseases, I may predict that it will cause a serious pandemic not milder than that caused by the swine flu (H1N1) in 2009 with more than 60 million cases and about 13000 deaths.
- Karine, is it you? You are always so optimistic. Why do you think so? - I hear from my colleagues and friends any time I try to explain the possible threats of the new coronavirus.

I have no proof of my words yet. This is a medical intuition, an experience, an opinion of experts in the field that are a minority so far. A lot of health care workers and public health authorities believe that it is a local infection only.

Everyone had a common cold at least once in his or her life. It is usually a mild illness of the upper respiratory tract resolving on its own within 1-2 weeks yet causing a huge impact on public health as one of the most frequent reasons for lost productivity and doctor visits. As a physician, I may list more problems due to the common cold. People often do not accept the fact that the common cold is an infectious disease caused by a variety of viruses, such as rhinoviruses, coronaviruses, adenoviruses, respiratory syncytial viruses, etc. There would not be any consequence of unacceptance of the viral origin of the common cold if it would not be contagious. When people admit and apprehend the infectious origin of an illness and its transmissibility, they will probably take action against it. These actions can be grouped in primary and secondary prevention; the terms indicating all effective measures to avoid contracting the illness, to defend others from being infected, and to prevent further complications, correspondingly. Without going deep into details, I will bring just a few examples of preventive measures against common cold: wearing masks; maintaining good air ventilation; staying at home when respiratory symptoms, such as cough, sneezing, nasal discharge, are present; frequent and proper handwashing techniques; improving general health and immune resistance. These are nonspecific actions reducing the chances of common cold and other respiratory infections to acquire and spread. There is also specific prevention, vaccines, available for many infectious diseases. However, the diversity of causative agents of the common cold do not allow scientists to create an effective vaccine able to cover all of them. Additionally, no rationale to invent a vaccine for a predominantly mild and self-limiting condition such as the common cold. Because of a variety of common cold viruses, the same person may become infected with another common cold virus right after recovery, a condition named reinfection. It can be mistaken as prolonged recovery or a bacterial complication. Even without reinfection, people do not like waiting for 10-14 days until symptoms resolve. Many of them tend to try useless and often harmful supplements and medications, like antibiotics. This is the ten million eighteen thousand three hundred forty-sixth time I talk about pointless and hazardous prescription of antibiotics.

- What is wrong with taking an antibiotic that kills the virus?
- If we refer to the word etymology, "antibiotic" means "against microbial life". Viruses, bacteria, fungi are examples of well-known microbes. So, antibiotics include antiviral, antibacterial, or antifungal medications. However, the first antibiotics revealed and then synthesized were antibacterials, therefore, traditionally saying "antibiotic" we understand an antibacterial agent. So, in this scope, antibiotic does not work against virus.
- So, why can't we take an antiviral for the common cold?
- There is no effective antiviral medication available for the treatment of the common cold.
- Why?
- For the same reasons explaining the absence of a vaccine against the common cold.
- What about Tamiflu?
- It is an antiviral medication, oseltamivir, effective against influenza virus., that is not a common cold, but a more severe respiratory tract infection.
- I have heard about cold medications and herbal supplements stimulating antiviral immunity or having direct antiviral potency. Which one would you advise?
- Neither one. They are not proven to be effective, despite the advertisement and fairy tales told. Furthermore, many of them may cause severe and sometimes unpredictable side effects. The other group of cold medications sold without prescription contains pain killers, antifebrile agents, and nasal congestion reducers and are used just for symptomatic relief.
- If a common cold is complicated with a bacterial infection, then antibiotics are the right choice?
- Bacterial superinfection manifesting with new or persistent symptoms of common cold, - is not so frequent, as it is supposed. When another

microorganism, in this case, the virus in the upper respiratory tract weakens local barriers and immunity, some strains of our normal inhabitants, so-called facultative pathogenic bacteria, have a chance to cause inflammation, such as sinusitis, otitis, bronchitis, etc. Even if this happens and we do not confuse common cold symptoms or a viral complication itself, antibiotics are not always necessary.

- So, how these activated bacteria can be resolved on their own?
- Let us not ignore the incredible work that our immune system performs.
- I still do not understand why it is incorrect to use antibacterials? Less active bacteria, less work to do for our immune system.
- Our organism, as well as our relationship with microbes is not so simple. The immune system is activated via microbes and their particles. Using antibacterials and even symptoms relievers, we may somehow blind the immune awareness. Additionally, bacteria are much elder habitants of the earth and undividable, essential part of us, outnumbering our cells by 10 to 1. Tell me would you fight against annoying flies and mosquitos by atomic bomb?!
- No, - my questioner answers laughing, - Fascinating! Could you tell me more, please?
- Nature does not like empty spaces. If we eradicate, kill or fight against one species, another, usually worse one, will fill in its place. We must weigh possible harms and benefits any time we prescribe or take antibiotics, as well as any other medication. Furthermore, there is another jeopardy - bacterial resistance against antibacterial medications. Any time we receive an antibiotic, especially the "wrong" one, that is not indicated for our condition; in the wrong dosage; for a shorter than indicated period; or whenever "we can take this virus no long" the bacteria living in our organism may develop resistance to the antibiotic.
- Yes, I know, Doctor Karine! Then the same antibiotic will not work on the same bacterium, - I receive the answer followed by the expected question, - On the same or another bacterium?
- Both scenarios are possible. As living organisms, microbes cooperate, especially within the same family. When you acquire a new bacterial infection, usually more pathogenic than what you have already had, your resistant bacterium or bacteria and the new one can exchange their genes, including resistance or susceptibility genes, in your organism. Even if the new bacterium was initially sensitive to the medication, now it becomes drug-resistant due to your "own" bacteria. Note that this is not only harmful to you. You can infect others with mutated and antibiotic-resistant bacterial infection with all its petrifying consequences. So, you see, we are bound with other chains of this world, and "we are responsible for those we tamed".

- Doctor, had you been prescribing a lot of antibiotics, - when you were in practice?
- Surprisingly, the opposite. I had been prescribing antibiotics the least among my colleagues. When I was a beginner, a lot of patients had been referred to me just for antibiotic prescription, most of them uselessly. Complaints here and there like "what kind of infectious disease doctor is she that does not prescribe antibiotics?" were predictable then. Slowly but surely my extra efforts were being justified with no complaints or poor outcomes of my patients.

I continue answering multiple questions that are still in the stage of simple curiosity, but not in the stages of "possible risks" or "self-protection and prevention". Anyway, I do my best in clarifying all misunderstandings and queries.

"In 2002 (please, do not try to find out numerological mysteries between 2002 and 2020, it is just a coincidence!) a coronavirus received higher than it was used to attention for the first time. Cases of severe atypical pneumonia consequently named severe acute respiratory syndrome (SARS) were described in Guangdong Province, China (again in China and again no mystery, just another coincidence!), and later spread via international travel to more than two dozen countries and caused global concern. Until now we have poorly understood issues linked with SARS, however, it demonstrated that animal coronaviruses could become transmissible from animals to humans. Specialists predicted that it could happen again with another coronavirus and possibly with wider spread and hazards. By the way, many microbes not only the coronavirus may jump the biological barriers between species, for instance, the influenza virus".

These kinds of explanations may seem pointless wasting my time, just history, or information one can read on the web if necessary. But I find them an important part of effective infection control. We need to talk and learn about microbes, their positive or negative gigantic impact on our lives. We can spend enormous time shopping, news about celebrities and stars, public events, and social media, but we are so naive to neglect microbes and even our health. I have nothing else against the above-mentioned activities. I say this rather with love than judgment. A lot of people even well-educated ones do not believe in natural processes and origins of infections, epidemics, and pandemics. They more readily accept antiscientific statements and directions, like "biological weapons", "punishment from heaven", "viruses do not exist, no one has seen them yet", "pulling the wool over the eyes", "dirty games of powers that be", "it is just a business". Everything is simpler than our minds can imagine. Surely, we are answerable for our mistakes and sins toward ourselves or others, still taking microbes into account as a punishment is not a productive way of thinking. On the opposite, it does not allow us to notice the effectiveness of small steps in their prevention, the wonders following our tiny efforts, everyone's role on this unique and powerful organism, the Earth.

As deeper, I dig into medical sciences and human organisms, as stronger I see the links and chains binding us together. Any one of us can make this world better, reduce the risks and results of global tragedies: wars, epidemics, suicides, divorces, spoiled children, homelessness, drug addiction... This list can be continued long. At the first sight, this may sound nonscientific and meaningless, but everything is easier than it seems. Just do what you do in its best manner thinking and caring for others. You are a student, a driver, a housewife, a parent, a businessman, a singer, a social media personality, a patient, a prisoner, a homeless, a physician, a governor, a traveler, you are alive, so you have the power to act, to dream about something great and meaningful being sure that you can accomplish it, to do something new and beautiful today, to say something nice and sincere to a stranger. No matter what but do it with love, care, and responsibility.

History is not just a collection of curious or, the opposite, boring facts. It is one of our best teachers. So, if we go eight years back, we will meet another highly pathogenic coronavirus. In 2012, a disease named Middle East respiratory syndrome (MERS) emerged, caused by another highly pathogenic coronavirus. In contrast with SARS, MERS was localized more in Saudi Arabia and was eliminated in a relatively short period showing mostly sporadic zoonotic, i.e., from animals to human transmission, and higher case fatality rate, the proportion of deaths from a concrete disease (approximately, 36% and 10% for MERS and SARS, respectively). Despite clinical and epidemiological differences between SARS and MERS, the coronavirus family illustrated the threat to public health. In 2017, World Health Organization (WHO) placed these two coronaviruses on its Priority Pathogen list to stimulate research and defensive measures development against them. However, now, in January 2020 we still do not understand what to expect from the new coronavirus and how to protect ourselves.

The United States and several other countries initiate entry screening of passengers from Wuhan at major ports of entry. In other Chinese cities, Thailand, Japan, and South Korea individuals are being isolated for further monitoring and care if they are identified as travel-related cases. On January 20, a young Chinese man who has visited Wuhan (returned from Wuhan on January 15, developed the disease on January 19) represents the first, travel-related case in Washington state. Everyone familiar with common epidemiological features of infectious, particularly, viral diseases, understands that this is the first but not the only case in the United States. For every single infectious disease, the number of identified cases is just the tip of the iceberg. It does not signify that the public health authorities or physicians fail their work. The explanation is in peculiarities of infections. The infectious diseases, despite the different levels of their transmissibility and fatality, have an incubation period. This is the timeframe, - when the causative agent has already entered the host organism and is being reproduced to reach the adequate level to cause pathological changes. Without reproduction inside the human organism, microbes would be conquered by our protective mechanisms. The incubation period of infectious diseases varies from hours to years and from individual to individual. If the disease is contagious, infected people, still having no symptoms, can spread the causative agent to others for the last days or hours of incubation period without being aware. Some percentage of infected people may not develop symptoms for the whole course of the infection. These people represent asymptomatic cases characteristic for any infectious disease, starting from frequent and self-limiting ones, such as common cold, ending with serious and chronic ones, like HIV infection. We may just guess the percentage of these asymptomatic or undiagnosed cases. Even though there are various laboratory tests able to diagnose asymptomatic cases, it is neither practical to try catching them all, nor cost-effective.

Precise or approximate case fatality or other rates, poor or good outcomes prognosis, risks of complications, and other numbers are what I always pay attention to but dislike the most in medicine. These are values used to describes processes in the population. However, as a practicing specialist who deals with an individual, I never know whether my patients or their relatives, me, or my beloved ones, will fall into small percentage or big. "The chances to recover from this disease are 5% or 95%" … Statements like this are very vague for a concrete patient sitting in front of me. Any time in a similar situation, I remember my biology teacher who said once "we do listen to weather forecasts, even so, we will know tomorrow's weather the next day after tomorrow". If numbers tell me there are no chances for my patient to survive, I must be honest with him or her as a doctor, meanwhile, I hope the recovery till the end, as a human.

Resuming January 2020, I can say the novel coronavirus (2019-nCoV) outbreak is not currently under control, with a high risk of spread globally. It is already morning, but a lot of people are still asleep deeply ignoring alarms and wake-up calls. As for me, I am awake working at home and expecting others to wake up. I am an infectious disease physician backstage who hopefully waits for the time to act.

February 2020

Going downhill without breaks

I enjoy my 10-15-minute stroller rides with Eddy. My health is being recovered and my independence is being reestablished via these rides. Now I may walk for shopping groceries at the closest supermarket and visit my parents-in-law leaving nearby. These are the only two places that I may "afford" myself without a driving license and with my husband being at work. This is all I need even though it sounds weird for the person who has been actively involved in the job, education, and social life a short time ago. Studying at a medical university with the highest grades; taking part in Olympiads and public activities; combining jobs at the hospital and university; being a part of a big friendly family; having a lot of hobbies compose just a partial list of my favorite things I was used to doing in Armenia. Now I am just a mom! Though it is the highest position that a woman may reach in this world: endless love and care, extreme responsibility, utmost feedback, and a 24/7 working schedule. Everyone who has been in the United States may understand how it is to live without driving, especially with an infant. You can do nothing, no doctor visits, no shopping, no groceries, no playgrounds… But I am a thankful person overjoyed for every visible or invisible, small or great, lost or gained thing in my life. I am happy having a healthy family, feet, a stroller for my baby, a supermarket, and parents-in-law within reach. Driver license, car, work permit, dreamed job, friends, hobbies…?! They will come into my life on time! Victor struggles at work 60-80 hours per week being at home briefly for some rest and sleep. When he is home, he helps me as much as he can stay awake. He cares for Eddy so gently and touching that I cannot help myself falling in love with him again and again. These minutes all together do not allow us not to miss each other yet are enough to exchange affectionate words and keep the fire turned on.

As a physician, I follow rapidly updating information on novel coronavirus. In a single-center case series hospital-related transmission and 4.3%, mortality is described. Compared with SARS and MERS, it appears lower although more easily contractible with the most frequent human-to-human mechanism of transmission. As of February 4, 2020, the novel coronavirus (2019-nCoV) has spread to at least twenty-six countries with overall 180 cases, including 11 cases in the United States. These facts signal the upcoming unpredictable involvement of the global population. China still faces a serious stage of the outbreak with about 20 000 cases that are 98.9% of all registered cases. The list of clinical features is still being corrected. It includes fever and upper airway congestion, clearer, difficulty breathing through the nose is the most frequent symptom reported. Cough, sore throat, myalgia, headache, and occasionally, diarrhea is also observed. According to another source, fever and dry cough are the most common symptoms: again, nothing specific in the clinical manifestation of the disease. There is a case described a 2-year-old patient with a one-week fever and two-week cough before 2019-nCoV diagnosis warranting more attention toward similar presentation in kids. What is general in these reports is that the disease is dominantly mild or moderate and the symptoms are not specific. They can be observed in many other non-viral and viral diseases. In the majority of cases of infectious diseases, physicians do not need to order diagnostic tests to clarify concrete viral etiology. We usually look at the whole picture: epidemiological data; seasonal features; a combination of these nonspecific symptoms, which of them is more prominent or appeared earlier; the duration of the disease; and so forth. This strategy is especially valuable in countries with limited resources. We typically use laboratory tests when the cases are serious and we need to make a precise diagnosis for specific etiological treatment, if available; or if there is an epidemiological threat.

I receive an offer to be a consultant in a medical center in Armenia. This is what I can do on distance with my valid Armenian license. I also can perform scientific work, thus, me and my friend of twenty years and a talented surgeon in Armenia, John, start research on patients with the novel coronavirus if one will address their clinic for surgical problems. The outbreak in China and its spread says nothing to a lot of specialists in various countries, but my medical intuition and knowledge tell me about the approaching storm we are not ready to resist. Meanwhile, at the end of February, there is not enough preparedness. Many sources still mention that the great attention toward coronavirus disease 2019 (COVID-19) is exaggerated and consider it just a limited outbreak. Instead, the ongoing severe influenza season is urged to attract more awareness as it has started with the Center for Disease Control and Prevention (CDC) estimated twenty-nine million ill people and 16 000 deaths. On February 27, 60 cases in the United States and no death cases are recorded, seemingly nothing serious. The Health Ministry authorities in Armenia also do not intend to take "the rumors about this more pathogenic than usually common cold" seriously. On the other hand, WHO declared a Public Health Emergency of International Concern regarding COVID-19 on 30 January 2020. These kinds of contrary attitudes pose questions and concerns that I receive even more than in January and elicit to my best.

Suddenly, I develop a sore throat and body ache for two days followed by hacking cough spells interfering with food intake and sleep. Almost simultaneously, my parents-in-law get similar symptoms along with a high fever for a week. Victor has a milder form of the disease. No symptoms are observed in Eddy may be partially due to breastfeeding. The infectious disease specialist speaks inside me. "So, this is a viral infection, a common cold, flu, adenoviral infection, or COVID-19. Rhinovirus is the most prevalent cause of the common cold, however, neither of us has well-expressed catarrhal symptoms. Cough like mine can be observed in whooping cough or Mycoplasma, but these options fall out considering my recent vaccination status and the disease presentation in other family members. Hence, this is probably COVID-19", - I conclude. I have no chance and indication to address to a doctor, though I advise my parents-in-law to call their doctor. They are instructed to do things we used to do during a common cold, i.e., staying hydrated, taking fever reducers, having rest, and going to the urgent care, if no improvement in 5-7 days or there is a new or worsening symptom. Consequently, we have no diagnosis, and I am counseled "to stop being a doctor at home".

Sleepless nights, viral illness, physical isolation, loneliness, either altogether, or something else lead to a drop in milk supply. Eddy stops gaining weight, - and is now bound to me almost permanently, waking up every hour at night for breastfeeding. And we need to be as calm as possible to let Victor have some refreshing sleep. I try to add the formula, Eddy refuses many formulas, many bottles. Nothing works for us to improve our mutually connected and worsening condition. I am lost and stressed perceiving myself as a terrible mother, a feeling that probably every new mommy has had at least once.

March 2020

Acceptance

During my carrier in Armenia, I had been studying psychology and psychiatry as an additional subject of interest as I found them important in becoming a professional and in figuring out the patients' hidden problems. So, I could successfully recognize subtle, atypical, or masked forms of depression in my patients, students, and friends and direct them to proper specialists. The shoemaker going barefoot! Exhausted with ineffective breastfeeding and increasing guiltiness, I address to a lactational specialist who helps me at least in ascertaining the postpartum depression. It has started subtly and has been missed out from my vision. The way of thinking of a new mom has been changed and the physician's brain has been blocked. Now I long to receive help myself instead of giving, but all the breastfeeding tips, pumping, formula-feeding trials, and other instructions preclude my therapy. After few days I finally manage to reach the pediatrician's office. Victor accompanies me and Eddy, both crying, me from emotional "overload", Eddy - from hunger. Thankfully, this time right there, in the doctor's office my sweetie takes the bottle. What a relief! In the upcoming days, I see Eddy restarts gaining weight. Now I can catch a breath and "enjoy" the benefits of mixed feeding. All is well that ends well! "So, does it worth talking about postpartum depression?! Is it suitable for me? Isn't it shameful? I love my baby! I have been dreaming of him for so long and I care for him with attention, love, and patience. I am well educated, enough strong woman. Even though I let the depression started, I can control it now on my own. Otherwise, I will be judged and misunderstood, so, it is better to hide inside", - I burden myself with these thoughts. How many women, new mommies may recognize themselves saying these words. How many of them would confess they did? I do not know exactly, though I can guess that too many. I am a person who would rather solve her problems alone, - than disturb others until I find the problem overwhelming. I try to involve as few people as possible. However, when the challenge is overcome, I tell and share the gained experience readily as I think it can be useful and motivating for other people in the same situation.

The statistics of the National Institute of Mental Health show 10-20% of new moms experience postpartum depression. The signs and symptoms are as follow:

- Restlessness, anger, or irritability,
- Sadness, crying a lot,
- Worthlessness or guilt,
- Fear of hurting baby or yourself,
- Overly worried about the baby or not concerned about the baby at all,

- Little or no energy,
- Headaches, chest pains, rapid heartbeat, numbness or tingling in the hands or feet, or fast and shallow breathing,
- Trouble sleeping well,
- Poor eating habits,
- Trouble focusing, remembering, or making decisions,
- Little interest in things you used to enjoy, including sex.

"Trouble sleeping well?", "Poor eating habits"?! Hard to imagine a new mom having time to sleep, to eat well, or to prepare healthy food. Me who has always adored veggies and fruits, - now can afford just very few of them, those requiring no time for clean and cutting. Among the above-mentioned symptoms I notice guilt for not having enough milk for my baby; having no time for sleep rather than the trouble of sleeping; eating ready and caloric food as a poor eating habit, and irritability manifesting as intolerance toward critics and unasked advice concerning Eddy's care.

A mild depression or baby blues is common in 50% of new moms. Other sources state that up to 75% develop any form of postpartum depression. Probably, close to 100%? Maybe the professionals in this field will offer another, reviewed criteria and a term that would be less judgmental yet able to "catch" all cases and threats posed by it. A new term for this "pretty common" condition, the condition that is not normal for surrounding people and professionals but quite natural for women who gave life to another human, whose organism transformed for nine months incredibly and continues transforming after delivery, whose life and responsibilities change crucially. Even if the new mom goes back to her job and her seemingly previous life soon after delivery, she still undergoes these huge changes with or without breastfeeding. Moreover, one in ten men pre-or postnatal depression is observed showing that the condition is not linked just with physiological changes. From my point of view, the most important points during mood swings, blues, and depression are acceptance, no self-blaming, talking out, an acknowledgment that there is always at least one person who will understand, support, and help to overcome this "abnormally normal" period. When talked out, many people will probably criticize, give useless or even hurtful advice, nevertheless, more supporting people will appear, as well. Additionally, the little human helps immensely with all the cute smiles, positivity, love, unblemished soul, and naiveness. Eddy makes me a better person, mommy, and a woman day by day! If there is at least one tiny seed of love, we will see that our babies, the little angels, come to this world to make it better. But, if sadly, there is no love, the opposite happens, the world turns them into evildoers, unhappy, unsuccessful, permanently offended, or lonely people. We are responsible for everyone, especially for every child. Even a little bad thing, a poor habit, a mild or unrecognized addiction, a nasty word said, a rule not obeyed influence negatively on them. Therefore, whatever we wish for our children starts with ourselves.

So, what happened with my postpartum depression? The lactational consultant was very friendly and offered me to join the mothers club once per week stating that it helps the most. I feel that mommy's club will work for me, I just need to talk out, to hear a little bit of supporting, "specific for new mommies" words that I have been receiving only from my sister Irina in Armenia who became a mom year earlier than me. I arrange my transportation and Eddy's care to attend the mommy's club, but it is canceled. Again, alone with my problem, this time unwillingly? I am not! I start to look at the situation from another scope. There is a little cute human with me, and he gives me the hugest emotional support and feedback. Since the moment of the postpartum depression acceptance, it is turned into a good life coach; an alarm to be less proud, to become braver and neglect the fear of being misunderstood or judged, to appreciate much more all the blessings I have in my life; to use all the life favors more efficiently and to ask for help more steadily. I share with Victor my "diagnosis", explain that there are things out of my control, that "I did not feed the depression". He understands, worries, hugs, and says, "You are an amazing mom and wife, you do great, even though I miss you being "completely mine". These words sound like a hint "Being a new parent is not that easy for both parents, but we will overcome everything". Instead of expecting more from him, I start seeing him overloaded and in a tense situation. I know well what it means to be torn between job and family, to try being successful in both beloved aspects, especially if the wage and job environment are not that good as expected. With these changes of my point of view, with more prayers, and hard work performed in my mind and soul, the postpartum depression disappeared as subtly as it appeared.

Meanwhile, multiple questions keep coming not only from the United Stated but also from Armenia, Russia, Israel, Iraq, India, Brazil, Germany, France, Uzbekistan, Holland, Switzerland, Australia. This is the geography of my relatives, friends, students, and colleagues. The questions mostly are about protective measures. "Is there a real danger to be afraid of?", "How we can protect ourselves", "I have recently had a common cold, do I have a protective immunity against COVID-19? ", "Do we need to wear masks? Indoors or outdoors? Do they protect?", "How often do we need to change the masks? Can we wash them?"," How to deal with the PPE shortage?", "Isn't it dangerous for general health to wear a mask so long?" "If the masks are effective in reducing the speed of transmission, isn't it better to let the infection spread at its own pace?" …

March 11, WHO declares COVID-19 pandemic, i.e., the epidemic occurring across the globe, or a very wide zones, crossing international borders. March 13, National Emergency is declared. On March 15, we move to a bigger house that is far from

Victor's parents, but we will have enough space for Eddy's growing demands and my workout routine, a proper kitchen to enjoy cooking delicious food for my lovely family. The situation with COVID-19 is changing drastically in the United States; by March 17, the outbreak is already not just several isolated clusters located in just three states (Washington, New York, and California), but it is already spread to all 50 states, indicating on the definitive community spread of the disease. March 19, we are still adapting to the new house, arranging, cleaning, buying new things; and the "Stay home Executive and Public Health Order" is given.

The questions become full of panic, complaints, hopelessness, intolerance, depression, and even aggression. "Impossible to stay within four walls, they seem squeezing me", "This is boring and overwhelming", "I cannot resist this anymore", "Why we need to obey nonsense rules, just risky groups should be in isolation", "This isolation makes me feel depressed and useless", "Some countries do not close borders, do not announce shutdown, even do not force wearing masks everywhere, but they have few cases of the disease. This is very suspicious", and so on, and so on.

The lockdown was announced later than it should be. Delayed preparedness! The pandemic is several steps ahead of our readiness, but the antiscientific explanations and conclusions are spreading so fast and are making professionals in the field drive crazy. Once I met our neighbor, a nurse at the hospital. She has not seen her 14-month-old daughter for days. Healthcare professionals struggling with enormous problems that are a topic for another book, however, some people far from the medicine blame them for "just doing their duties", "earning money", "lying for their benefits", "killing patients", etc. My patience and understanding help me to weaken these kinds of opinions as I am a physician backstage. My current functions are educating people, explaining scientific and objective approaches, ensuring whenever possible, and trying to protect colleagues from attacks and wrong blames.

As for me, this lockdown did not change my life. Indeed, I have been in "lockdown" for more than a year. I know quite well what people feel now. For the reason of my overstay as a tourist in the United States and some other circumstances, my status legalization has been delayed. When I have been asking other immigrants in different countries how long it took them to adapt to a new life, they mentioned various periods, from six months till eight years, most of them – two years. Being stuck at home with almost no interaction with other people, a year seemed me a decade. I have been missing my parents, sisters, relatives, friends, medicine, my jobs, patients, students, my style, even sleepless nights in the hospitals, challenging situations when I needed to act fast and precisely. Now when a lot of people all over the world encounter a similar situation yet for few days, I share my experience with deep sympathy to encourage and comfort them. "How were you dealing with all of this?" – they keep asking me. In brief, by living now and here, by being thankful for the past and the present, by belief in upcoming great accomplishments, by love, patience, and faith. Changing the attitude and pointing out the positive sides existent in every situation, many problems and negativity are resolved. One can be in physical isolation but be loved more than another one surrounded by many people who pay no attention to each other. I already used to see my relatives and friends via phone and to be thankful for the opportunity, as I am from that generation who saw the first phone with cables at the age of seven. It was the neighbor's telephone, the only one for several families. Later when we finally obtained our own and fix it on the wall, I used a ladder to climb, dialed our phone number to see if someone would pick it up or no. My first cellphone, an old Motorola with a black and white screen and no internet, I received from my sister Irina as a gift in my fourth year of medical university. In case if you are curious, I am not so old to have a chance to see dinosaurs! It is the technical and scientific progress that develops rapidly.

The "Stay Home Order" probably made a lot of people suffer but did a favor to me. Now I may see Victor at home, even though I know very well how frustrating and torturing staying at home can be for him. Thankfully, in the United States, people receive financial support and compensation for unemployment. There are countries where this was told but did not work in practice. However, I think that the heaviness of the problem is never stronger than one's shoulders can carry. On the third day of lockdown with all the spare time available, I, who adores studying and reading every day, persuade Victor, who is capable to learn easily but hates reading and writing, to admit a college. His dislike toward reading has resulted in many funny family stories. Once our toothbrushes happened to be the same color and form, so I took a nail polish to write our initials on them.

- What are you doing, Karine? -Victor asked me.
- Writing our names, - I answered surprised by his question.
- Why write?
- Hmm, because I adore writing, - I said laughing.
- Better to bind a thread on it! You like writing, but me, I hate reading!

Now, I propose to him an incredible thing, to study something new at a college. Surprisingly, he accepts my proposal readily and even offers the profession of medical biller and coder. "This is what I am interested in and can do to be closer to you when you restart medicine", - he explains. Honestly, I have not heard about this profession before. Then he adds, - "But you have to help me with studying". With pleasure! As much as I love studying, I also adore teaching. So, he enters a college. The minimum length of education for the profession is four months that can be prolonged to one year. There are many private classes and training for medical billers and coders, but we decided to receive the education at the highest possible level. So, now the boring and depressing lockdown becomes a fun family time. Victor listens to his auditory books, watches educational videos, then I explain medical terms, diagnosis, and other hard parts. We create a puzzle to combine Latin word parts and to compose medical terms. Eddy who received an intrauterine highest medical education preparing and passing my USMLE Step 3 during the pregnancy, has a lot of fun with us and turns Victor's tortures into a family-pleasant entertainment. I remember when I was studying anatomy and histology at the medical university, we were drawing from the books, posters, and even from microscopic specimens. I keep those notebooks; one day they may appear in a museum! Educating people online, helping Victor with his studies, seemed not sufficient to me. So, I also started learning my fifth and sixth foreign languages, Spanish and Hebrew. Why these languages? Spanish is spoken in more than twenty countries, - and is derived from Latin, a dead language nowadays used just in medicine and religion, so, it is easy for me to learn. As a second language in California, it is also useful. Hebrew may seem a strange choice as it is spoken just among Jews but I have liked it since I traveled with daddy to Israel. While listening to it, I feel being again in Israel with my father. The absence of written vowels makes it challenging and interesting. My friends ask how I find time for them with my family duties, workout routine, online job, and rest. Easy! It is a kind of rest. Funny and effective applications 30 minutes per day are much better than news or selfies on social media. Is it possible to learn a new language like this? It is! Every drop counts!

Meanwhile, the COVID-19 pandemic evolves quickly. I have experience working during respiratory infection pandemics, but this one, as I see it, is much worse. In 2009-2010 during the influenza pandemic, I was a second-year fellow of infectious diseases at the only specialized infectious disease hospital. A second-year fellow in Armenia still works under the supervision but is no longer a beginner, has maturing self-confidence, enough rich knowledge, a lot of courage, and enthusiasm. Features suitable for the pandemic! Armenia is a small country, so the republican hospital of infectious diseases can be described as one having about 200-bed capacity. Qualified is equal to super interesting, challenging, and difficult cases, that could not be solved in primary chains. Within thirty-month of my job there (rather education as fellows receive no wages in Armenia!), I have seen so many interesting cases that many professionals can hardly meet during the whole carrier: leishmaniosis, leptospirosis, brucellosis, malaria, anthrax, tularemia, and "other petrifying words" – not the full list. Since my first days of residency, as an outstanding graduate, I had been receiving a lot of "benefits"; allowed to work in departments where no other residents were working; having night-shift duties at six departments simultaneously instead of three, as other fellows were doing; taking part in the educational process, such as teaching medical students; creating guidelines and handbooks. I was happy with these "advantages" because of the great chance to learn as much as I could. When the H1N1 pandemic started, I started volunteering in the most overloaded department – the military department. Hundreds of patients during each shift. Additionally, military service had its peculiarities and rules. It required me to be more organized, strict, and act rapidly. Military patients could not be sent back "home" for observation or home recovery. It was tough to bridge the gap between job and family. I was going home just to change clothes and to have some refreshing sleep. My family – parents, and sisters, became used to my absence. Once, while I slept in my room, a friend of mine came to visit me. And when she asked about me, they forgot that I was home sleeping and said, "she is at the hospital as always". Another time, on my father's birthday, when the pandemic was going down, I went home exhausted but happy from our results and recovering patients. I sat on the sofa in the living room for a refreshing 15-minutes nap, as I was used to doing, - while waiting for the guests. When I woke up from the nap, I realized that it was almost midnight, all the guests came and went, the birthday party was over. I slept the whole birthday being a nice decoration for the living room furniture. I know like the back of my hand how heroic are all healthcare professionals in the frontline during this pandemic. Hats off to them all!

Now when I go for a walk with Eddy, I see the fear on neighbors' faces, the fear of being infected, the fear of vagueness. This is war! Nothing else might shut down the heavy traffic of Los Angeles, the never-sleeping city. Humor is one of the psychological protective mechanisms. Many funny cartoons appear on social media: "exhausted pets being taken for a walk by each family member many times just to breath some air and see some sun", "family members who find out each other quite interesting persons after being forced to sit at home together", "online education and background family scenes". It would be fun… but people are dying. The majority, even my husband, say that this is not a real infectious threat, but "exaggerated" numbers. Now the facts and my explanations have no sense for them. "If it is so deadly, why we do not know anyone who died from it or at least was infected", - they tell me each time. Sadly, I know this is just a matter of time.

April 2020

The mountain with an invisible peak

What we currently know is that this pandemic develops like the disease itself: initially, it is mild and nonspecific, but several days later many patients attend to emergency departments with respiratory failure and worsening conditions. We do not know the exact real number of cases, hence, still no precise case fatality rate. It is varying widely by location from 0.7% reported in Germany to 10.8% in Italy. The average value is 4.7%, higher than that reported in the United States (1.7%).

Panic, anxiety, uncertainty, loneliness, apartness, financial crisis, fear, stagnation, not the full list of "side effects" of the lockdown. On the other side of the scales, there are courage, self-sacrifice, team battles, love, respect, support, faith. I felt on my skin that even wearing a mask 95 requires a huge effort. What to say about healthcare workers' tortures of fighting with a much stronger enemy, being sleepless, exhausted, detached from their families and beloved ones, forced to make tough decisions. Till this point, the feeling of uselessness as a professional, job nostalgia, and desire for a better new job in the United States had visited me not once. Now I understand the precious life gift I have by my documents being delayed. The problem we have been trying to resolve turns into a unique occasion, a favor allowing me to be next to my husband and our son, to see him growing day by day. I start loving him even more instead of all medical professionals in the frontline who do not have a chance to be with their kids. It may sound selfish at first sight, but I find meaning in any obstacle happening in my life.

Since the first case at the end of January, in more than 2 months over 235 000 cases (about one-fifth of global total cases) have been diagnosed and more than 5000 COVID-19-associated deaths have been registered across the United States. As in every infectious disease, especially fast-spreading ones we assume that the true number is likely much higher. The United States is now the number one country with the prevalence of COVID-19. This fact rises comments annoying me despite my huge patience and diligence.

- If the United States cannot fight the disease, no other country can. So, all these shutdowns, masks, social distancing are futile. - Ah, this is not too much for a country with more than three hundred million population.
- My dear followers, this is a real war threatening everyone in this world! Humans are dying! In another country or at your next door, - I stop talking as a physician. - Death is a loss for all of us despite nationality, race, ethnicity, age, comorbidities, or any other "difference". Some people can make a tragedy

having a favorite earing lost or a nail broke, people who spend money on evanescent things trying to fill in the void in their life ignoring others who may become happy with few pennies. Some people would not be so upset even losing money or a house, because these are just a staff. Today you have them, tomorrow - no, and the opposite. But when we speak about human beings, how can we compare or define which death is a less tragedy, which one - bigger?! No how. The coping mechanisms can be different during bereavement, even so, every life matters because we are the cells of the same alive organism named Earth.

I do not know how many people will stop and think over these words, but the posts and comments like these ceased at least on my page. Another storm of questions pops up from all corners of the globe.

- Can patients become reinfected?
- The pandemic is still brief and diagnostic methods are neither fully accurate nor conclusive for reinfection. There are cases described from China and Japan indicating hospital readmission of patients with positive swab real-time polymerase chain reaction (RT-PCR) results after initially negative ones at the time of discharge. However, it is not enough information to disclose the real reinfection as the negative results during discharge could be false negative. Theoretically, the reinfection may happen and probably in lesser severity due to at least partial immunity, but how long after the primary infection is still a big question to be solved. Additionally, as in all microbes, especially viruses, we cannot forget about mutability, so even if postinfectious immunity is strong and long-lasting, the virus may mutate and cause quite a severe reinfection, almost like a new virus. As you see, even professionals yet have tons of unclear concerns.
- So, no information on how long does the postinfectious immunity last and how strong it is?
- Yes. Just a few months of the epidemic do not allow us to judge postinfectious immunity. If we refer to SARS-CoV1 data, as another representative of the coronavirus family with some shared characteristics of the novel coronavirus, we can see that the level of neutralizing antibodies peaks at 4 months after infection and declines subsequently during at least 3 years after infection. Nonetheless, the titer of neutralizing antibodies is not a precise and complete indicator for postinfectious immunity, particularly, concerning viral infections. There are more important and not routinely analyzed indicators, such as cells that kill the virus and cells that produce the antibodies against the virus long after primary infection.
- Who should wear a mask?

- I may answer based on current guidelines from the CDC that do not recommend healthy individuals to wear masks routinely limiting mask use to health care workers, symptomatic individuals, and those caring for patients with COVID-19. Priority should also be given to people with the risk of exposure and development of a severe form of the disease. Though we are required to be watchful for any update on these guidelines and local authorities' orders.
- So, it means that I have not to wear a mask, haven't I?
- Not exactly. Rather we still do not have precise information on routine mask wearing for everyone while in public, as the current guidelines are based on data concerning influenza indicating limited efficacy of masks in protecting healthy individuals. Another argument upholding the recommendations is the need to preserve supplies for health care workers and other above-mentioned people groups. But we need to be aware of possible subclinical and asymptomatic forms of the disease, as well as about healthy individuals who can be at the end of the incubation period feeling well, having no symptoms yet, but already being a source of the infection. Additionally, washing hands with wearing a mask is more effective than either of them.
- How does the novel coronavirus spread?
- What we know about SARS-CoV-2, earlier 2019-nCoV, transmission in the community, is primarily via air droplet, larger particles (larger than aerosols) emitting from infected people while sneezing, coughing, breathing, talking. They can reach at least a 6 ft (1.8m)-distance. Transmission via aerosols is more common at hospitals, inpatient services where respiratory support and cardiopulmonary resuscitation are provided. Although spread through aerosols may happen in the community, as well, and probably, even to a greater extent than via air droplets. If this suggestion is taking place, the risk of contracting the infection is higher even with ideal social distancing and mask-wearing.
- Why do you think aerosols can be the most frequent way of transmission even in the community?
- This is not just my opinion. There are no precise data on this, but cases of many people who were following isolation firmly but were infected could be explained in this way.
- What are the sites of entry of this coronavirus?
- Respiratory mucosa and conjunctiva.
- Conjunctiva? Can it cause eye problems?
- Conjunctiva can serve as just a site of entry; however, eye involvement can also be observed. There is still not enough information on the direct or indirect mechanism of eye affection in COVID-19.

- What about surrounding objects? Can they be a source of the infection?
- The virus can remain alive on inanimate surfaces at room temperature for up to 9 days, shorter at greater than 86°F (30°C). Cleaning and disinfection decrease contamination of surfaces. Whether catching the disease via these contaminated inanimate objects is factual and in what amount is again an unresolved topic.
- If there are more questions than answers, why do we need to pursue social distancing? It is boring and depressing.
- New data are being updated from all over the world as faster as possible. Meanwhile, everyone must follow the established rules that help to reduce the speed of the pandemic and decrease the burden on healthcare systems.
- How long the lockdown will last?
- We may assume at least one-two years in less or stronger extent until the virus can become controllable.
- When will a vaccine be available?
- Only 3 vaccine candidates are currently in human trials. The estimated timeline for the availability of an initial vaccine is between early and mid-2021.
- What about the new symptom? If someone develops a loss of smell, it means coronavirus infection?
- Not obligatory. Anosmia, loss of smell, have many reasons, the most common ones (22-36%) - upper respiratory tract infections, such as common cold and influenza. However, anosmia described in coronavirus infection may happen even without signs and symptoms of upper respiratory tract infection, such as nasal obstruction or runny nose. Therefore, during this pandemic sudden anosmia with no other explanation can be an indication to test for the coronavirus.

When news about gastrointestinal and dermatological manifestations of the disease spread, many people started to tease and make fun saying "Now no one will have undiagnosed sickness. Every symptom will be attributed to coronavirus". With all mistakes, omissions, over-or under diagnostics, and unsettled issues in medicine, it is unfair to devalue every effort, every single recovered health, and a saved life. Describing multiple signs and symptoms observed in coronavirus infection, we do not forget about other diseases and infections. We do know that various other viruses may cause multiple organ involvement with a constellation of many symptoms, but lately, we talk mostly about COVID-19 because it is a new and ongoing illness affected 167 countries (as of April 11), and updating features are being reported for further investigations.

- If a healthcare worker is pregnant, she should refrain from work with patients?

- There are no general recommendations for pregnant medical professionals. As till now the information on possible outcomes of coronavirus infection for pregnant women and their babies is scarce, it is recommended to transfer them to another job without direct contact with suspected or diagnosed patients with COVID-19, - I respond and immediately contact my friend in Israel. She is a therapeutist who had an unexplained first-trimester loss of previous pregnancy and now works at a busy hospital in her second month of a third pregnancy. These last days she has been ready to quit her job, if necessary, to protect her developing baby. I am relieved to hear that she is transferred to do paperwork and organizational duties.
- Are there any extra precautions for the elderly or people with the coexisting disease? - another vulnerable question follows.
- The list of comorbidities is being updating, meanwhile people aged 65 and older; those with common chronic morbidities, like cardiovascular disease, diabetes, obesity, and arterial hypertension, better limit shopping or other contacts to the utmost. As more people and longer contacts, as higher the risk to get ill with coronavirus infection.

I educate people about the management of these comorbidities, the necessity, or the uselessness of revising their treatments. I exhort to follow healthy habits as primary and secondary prevention. However, I cannot persuade my 68-year-old father to limit his activities and shopping for groceries. He tries to limit the visits, nevertheless, staying at home and being isolated is hard for him. He used to do many things for our big family in Armenia. One of the caring and kind men there has ever been! After his early and unfair retirement, he has been supporting us even more: taking grandchildren to school, various training, trips; working at his garden to supply us, our relatives, and friends with delicious and organic fruits for the whole year; making all groceries. Being an early bird, he has been preparing coffee and breakfast while his beautiful daughters have been getting ready for work. Three years ago, on my parents' marriage forty-second anniversary I received my USMLE step 1 score report and was about to visit my parents with this gift. My father beat me visiting in the apartment where I had been isolated for the USMLE preparation and that was on the way from dad's garden to our home. With a long harvesting day under the sun, he was tired and hot. When he took off his T-shirt, I noticed petechiae and bruises on his back and arms. Perfectly knowing his character of hiding problems, I started asking him gentle and detailed questions but received escaping responses. Later Irina told she noticed him catching breath when climbing the trees or heights in the garden. Alarmed and worried, I persuaded him to run a proper analysis. After long and unbearable days, we finally found out his diagnosis: idiopathic aplastic anemia, severe form. This was like thunder in the clear sky. For my non-medical readers, I would explain aplastic anemia means bone marrow stopped producing blood cells, resulting in anemia with signs of hypoxia (shortness of breath, intolerance of physical activity, dizziness, and even life-threatening conditions, such as heart attack), low coagulation with bleeding risk under the skin, outside of the body, or inside the inner organs, for instance, brain (stroke); and leukocytopenia, i.e., absence of immunity. Idiopathic signifies "no reason established". And the disease has just two forms, severe and very severe. Soon after the diagnosis, he developed retinal hemorrhages, thankfully resolved in upcoming days, otherwise, they could lead to partial or complete blindness. The only treatment offered in Armenia was continuous blood transfusions with a prognosis of 6-12 months maximum. But with each blood transfusion, his condition was worsening. I saw in his eyes he was ready to give up partially due to pitiful glances from every corner. After long consultations with foreign colleagues and putting on a scale his chances, condition, expenses, visa requirements, the time we had, I took him to Israel. Bone marrow transplantation was canceled weighing possible risks and benefits. The medications giving us good chances to survive and even recover were not affordable for us. I addressed many charitable foundations and received similar answers. - "We preferably help younger people with better prognosis". No one to blame! Me, being a successful physician saving others' lives, was unavailing for my dad. We ended up with the administration of a single affordable medication that was available also in Armenia. The prognosis with only it was 50/50. If after two months no improvement is observed, it is generally being canceled, and the patients are being left "to live as long as they will". When we returned home to Israel, I was blamed for spending the family budget on "the same thing that could be done here". Even so, I was sure of my decision made. There in Israel, we enjoyed each other do our best, we went to the sea several times. I wrote on the beach far from waves "My dad is healthy" and saw his smile first time after an endless period of hardship. We met my friends who gave us so much hope, support, and care. Unforgettable days… When you face a dead-end and see no solution, try to make a trip. It can change or save lives! Daddy's medical condition was stabilized, and his mood was improved in Israel. After two months of no improvement, we were offered to stop the therapy. As I was administered by daddy "the responsible person for all his medical decisions" since the first day of the disease, I persisted in prolongation because I noticed he was feeling more confident with "some therapy than nothing". His disease started to regress. After a year, no blood transfusions were indicated, and he was a practically healthy man just "swallowing magical pills daily". This was a miracle! His caregivers were asking him whether his physician daughter gave him something else than the medication. Once I asked him what helped him to recover, he responded to me - "Your faith in my recovery!".

Now, the coronavirus, already overloading all over the world, poses another threat to his life. And this time I am far from him…

This month I cannot contact any of my colleagues in the frontline despite their geographical location. They have neither time nor energy for calls or messages. They just scramble the height without knowing ahead what to expect and how high to go. More than 500 deaths among healthcare workers worldwide as of April 2020! Overwhelmed with excessive work, often outside of their scope, for the same pay; hazarding themselves and their beloved ones; burned out emotionally and physically from hard decisions, losses, uncertainty, they are warriors and should be loved, cared for, and respected! Nevertheless, I observe attacking, aggressive and antiscientific opinions toward them. In the shadow of primary fighters, my job as the educator surprisingly appears successful. My statements and explanations are accepted by people! A small victory backstage!

May 2020

Fallen but not broken

It has been four months since I got the viral infection and have been suffering from the hacking cough. I have been prescribed an inhaler with no improvement. And now I develop tooth pain. The stomatologist has revealed the indication of wisdom teeth removal. After the procedure, antibiotics for ten days have been administered. On the 7th day, I have had to stop it because of nausea, severe abdominal pain, and rash. The steroids prescription follows with the improvement of all symptoms including the cough. Resolved cough with no diagnosis. I assume that it was a coronavirus infection. When I start asking people in the Los Angeles area, I revealed about twenty possible COVID-19 cases in February among my acquaintances. Neither much; nor precise, even so, if an infectious diseases physician, currently not in practice and with limited socialization, suspect twenty cases, most likely the real COVID-19 numbers are much higher than are being diagnosed.

At the end of May, I read in one of the most prestigious medical journals that the community spread of SARS-CoV-2 in the United States presumably took place earlier than thought and started from the sole traveler from China. The first two non-travel-related cases were just first detected but not the first ones. The United States Centers for Disease Control and Prevention COVID-19 Response Team reports that the virological analysis of the early cases indicated that the single virus type entered directly or indirectly into the United States from China between January 18 and February 9. This is what we, specialists in the field, guessed beforehand, in February. The first two California residents diagnosed with COVID-19 died on February 6 and February 17. They seemed to be the sources of virus circulation in California state by early February. Another opinion of an infectious disease specialist at the Johns Hopkins Center for Health Security expresses the same idea: there were cases in Europe in December 2019. Hence, we understand that a similar situation happened not just in the United States, but also in many other countries. If national preparedness systems would be reacted earlier and wider, not limiting on entrance prohibition of travelers, screening and testing only people who visited China recently, being more alert to all cold and flu cases (because of nonspecific general and overlapping symptoms of these viral infections), we would probably have a better situation. Yes, this is true, we want to hear it or no. We, people, not Americans, Europeans, Chinese, or others, not just health care authorities, but each of us, we unwillingly lost the initial battle with the virus. No one to blame, rather learn lessons. With technical and scientific progress, we forgot that humans are not the owners of the world, but just a respected part of it. There were, are, and will be stronger organisms than us once in a while to make us wiser, more patient, more modest, more loving, and more thankful.

This month my job profile does not change much. The new and most frequently asked question is about social distancing, its effectiveness, necessity, and possible extension or shortening of the "Stay home" order. I share the results of the investigations indicating that social distancing does flatten the curve of COVID-19 cases. This is hard to accept as we want the bans and restrictions to over faster. It is very tough for everyone. I do not remember any other similar period faced in the world. People need encouragement, empathy, explanations. I have talked about my isolation previously and it appears motivating and comforting others.

- This is what we experience right now just the fear of catching the virus added, - they comment. -How were you facing it? Watching TV, going to breathe fresh air, watching beautiful American landscapes?

- Sad to say, that the weather in Las Vegas was hot for me then. I had to wake up too early as the early morning was the only proper time to breathe some fresh air, enjoy the sun, the sky, the birds. I would like to say that TV was my only friend then, but it was not true. At first, I found it mostly useless. With the variety of channels and possibilities, there were just extremely limited programs I would watch and few movies I could find out after spending more time on the search than the movie itself. So, TV was (and still is!) a part of furniture to take the dust off. Even if I would be a TV lover, I could not afford me spending time on it. I was preparing for the USMLE Step 3 that took much longer than expected due to my pregnancy. Initially, I was irresistibly sleepy with almost no energy. Then when I regained my energy, I had to restrict my physical and emotional activity because of high-risk pregnancy that later, after the exam, resolved on its own. Additionally, the "cloudy" and shrunk brain of pregnancy played its role: forgetting in few minutes what I had just read and understood. But all these difficulties were not stronger than my will to pass the exam while I was expecting. I knew ahead that it would be impossible to do with a newborn. Plus, it was filling lapses and making my isolation meaningful. Any time I was reading a case presentation to solve, I imagined a real patient in front of me. Then, I pretended that studying is my job and the office room – my workplace. So, every morning after the walk I was going to the second floor, "the home", taking shower, preparing myself, and descending to the first floor, "the workplace". No driver's license is needed!

- It is fun and motivating, doctor, - everyone tells me any time I share my story.

- I am glad to hear. A little bit fantasy and you will find some interesting and useful entertainment for you. And let me add that now you are not in forced isolation, rather you are a soldier protecting others!

The lockdown is a good chance to realize things for what we have never had time. To enjoy our families or ourselves if living alone, to recover the missed time, to invent something interesting for all family members or to explore something new, a hobby, a skill, a new profession. There are so many options. Even though the hard time is in its full bloom, let us appreciate everything we have now and do not accept them for granted.

I and Victor receive the announcement from the lawyer that my paperwork is postponed due to a pandemic. This means another missed year for medical residency. When you expect something too much, it runs away from you! "I am going to forget everything I learned, I will be lost as a professional within an additional year!" – this kind of thought comes into my head. I find my potential as an unused treasure, like owing a Bugatti but driving it just in a garage. Few days pass. I start to realize how silly it is to lay down and spit on the ceiling. Getting back some wisdom, I remember about my reproductive potential. Victor, the best husband in the world, shares my desire to have another baby despite the challenging period, pandemic, and many other concerns. My father supports me, as well.

- Do not be afraid! I will come to take care of your children when you start to work, - he said full of decisiveness.
- Dad, how would you leave mom, the grandchildren, your garden, your trees? They are also like your children.
- Hmm, aren't you my child and your kids my grandchildren, too? – he joked and added, - I organized everything, Irina with her husband and my brothers will care of the garden while I am absent. No worries. Be brave and do what your heart tells you!

June 2020

Another month survived!

In June established COVID-19 cases among my acquaintances have already occurred. Most of them - compliant mask wearers. This raises another wave of misunderstanding.

- It is so unfair, no one else was wearing a mask, washing hands, and disinfecting as I was doing, but I got sick. I will not follow any rules further. I was air deprived with the masks for so long, changed them every two hours, as indicated, but I caught the virus. Now I must be in this torturing isolation and suffer from the disease.

- I am sorry you are facing it. I understand your frustration about the masks that seemed not to work. If you let me, I will clarify that the masks are not full protection against the infection, they rather decrease the chance of contracting it, as well as suppress transmission to others in case if one is contagious. The exact effectiveness level of masks is being investigated, as we still do not know whether transmission via air droplets or aerosols is predominant. Additionally, there can be a misunderstanding in wearing masks and "Stay Home" orders. A lot of people guess if they are compliant with proper face-covering rules, they have a guarantee and may go everywhere, for example, shopping. There are data about multiple contacts' role in COVID-19 transmission. I name it "the rule of fifteen". If you talk to an infectious person for about fifteen minutes even with masks, you can be infected by him or her. Or if you contact fifteen infectious persons for less than one minute during a day, again you are at high risk. So, as more people you meet per day and the longer the contacts, especially indoors, as higher your risk to be infected. By the way, an infectious person does not obligatory mean someone with fever or evident catarrhal symptoms, such as runny nose, sneezing, and coughing. You never know who is behind the mask! As you see, you did your best, yet were at risk of contracting the virus.

This month few of my friends in the United States tell me they struggle with the preparation for the registered nurses (RN) exam. One of them failed twice and is about to give up. Another one has been trying to combine her job at the hospital, her family of five, and RN exam. The others graduated abroad with a huge difference in the education program. Despite practice in their homelands, they try to become nurses in the United States. This is like a perfect bicyclist given a plane to fly for the first time. Overall, I find five nurses who need help. As I have enough knowledge, teaching skills, and some spare time, I decide to train them. For this purpose, I start to study the program myself. Thankfully, I learn a lot of new things, especially procedural and organizational, I get familiar with peculiarities of nurses' work in the United States that I do not know due to lack of practice here. I even passed the self-assessment exams with 80-90% of achievement. In a nutshell, I enjoy everything linked with medicine.

A new topic is added to my responses list: COVID-19 in infants and children. Cases are describing prolonged and severe complications in children with multiorgan involvement, similar to Kawasaki disease. Again, not a unique feature for SARS-CoV2. There are infectious and noninfectious agents that can cause likewise illness. But, in the majority of infants and children despite higher viral quantity in the nasal cavity, the disease's presentation is milder than in older children, adolescents, and adults. I notice an analogy in our daily life. Little kids take things easier than us. They may cry and forget the reason in a few seconds smiling through tears and filling our souls with love. They may be offended and forgive in no while. We can try to be a little bit like kids with their clear hearts and the way they look at the world. It would help us overcome easier this challenging period.

This month I receive a lot of positive feedback. My explanations and the way of resolving panic waves give a good harvest. I do it with all responsibility and, surely, for free. Though as in every single job, I receive also attacking messages. The one followed my clarification of the uselessness of the forced double isolation in asymptomatic people retested positive after 14 days of COVID-19. "You contribute to spreading the infection. People with the positive test result, and even the individuals with postinfectious established immunity, should stay at home until vaccines are available", - a healthcare worker explains to me. I answer, - "If you consider the postinfectious immunity too unstable and nonprotective, haven't you thought how vaccines will work and protect people or contribute to herd immunity? Isn't it futile to expect that vaccine will activate the immune system more than the disease itself?". Then I share the links of trustable sources I have been receiving daily. No more similar messages followed. Another person indicated to me to do my responsibilities as a homemaker and do not disturb people who work. Once I was also blamed for being "neither from Armenia; nor from the United States", to which I responded with humor "Yeah, - because I am a star living in the sky". The attacks ceased!

Many concerns come from the family members of individuals with comorbidities over and over, - "What to do with my vulnerable parents, grandparents, parents-in-law, husband, wife…? How to protect them?".

People with more than one risk factor are at the highest risk of being hospitalized. For instance, individuals with rheumatic and musculoskeletal diseases aged older than 65 years are five times more likely to be hospitalized and even more if prior use of glucocorticoids and accompanying cardiovascular disease. This poses suspicion to receive the treatment or cease it. The same situation was with one of the most commonly prescribing and effective antihypertensive medications – the angiotensin-converting enzyme group (lisinopril, enalapril, ramipril, perindopril, captopril, etc.). Even though this is not a primary subject of infectious diseases, but as long as it is linked with the coronavirus, I share all updates with my readers and followers indicating the uselessness of cessation or change of these medications (antihypertensives, steroids) while on them and if they work efficiently. Many people have a constellation of accompanying diseases, such as cardiovascular disease and hypertension, diabetes and obesity, or any other combination of them with or without other risk factors, such as advanced age. When I talk about this theme, I become one of the most vulnerable people in the world. Family, parents, children, our beloved ones, next of kin are our treasure, our way to heaven, our oasis during starvation and storms, our power, and our weakness! Not only my father is in the risk group, but my mother, too. She is 74 years old with hypertension, myocardial infarction with two stents, diabetes, and obesity. Medical ethics tell us not to diagnose or treat family members or friends. I agree! Nevertheless, it happened that I diagnosed her illnesses starting from my student years. I was a fourth-year student who recently started a job at one of the best hospitals in Armenia as a laboratorian on duty with frequent night shifts. In 2006 in my country, it was almost unacceptable when a young girl, especially a student who "just need to study", works at night. It was too hard to combine the job with the highest achievements at the medical university, but I was happy for that chance to work at the hospital and to receive a huge experience that was insufficient with just education. My professors noticed in me a good medical intuition I had no idea about. That night I was on duty and missed my niece's birthday party. In the morning when I came home, I saw an ambulance leaving our building. Reaching home, I revealed that my mom had developed abdominal pains and vomiting soon after the party, i.e., eating cake and fruits. She was diagnosed with food poisoning by the physician of the ambulance, had her stomach pumped at home, and nothing else. No comments here! I found her weak and drowsy, because of "sleepless night and dehydration". I organized her analysis and revealed remarkably high blood glucose levels enough for the initial diagnosis of diabetes. She had almost no symptoms before this episode. She was shocked and could not believe I found out and "impose" this diagnosis on her. Stereotypes harm people! She had been hearing so many horror stories about diabetes… Only after two weeks, I persuaded her to go to an endocrinologist for full diagnostics and treatment. Since then, she had been managed properly for her diabetes and accompanying hypertension. In 2018, after several weeks of coming-going abdominal pains, she developed intractable vomiting. She was taken to the hospital by me, undergone gastroscopy with biopsy, and received the initial diagnosis of gastric cancer. I wish no one to face that kind of situation. A few years ago, we lost our aunt because of duodenal cancer. A kind, brave woman full of love and energy! Her family decided not to disclose her diagnosis being afraid that she could not accept it and could try to commit suicide. As the only physician in all our great kinship, she kept asking me questions about her diagnosis and prognosis. I had to lie and hated myself for that. She had also chronic gastritis and cholecystitis for many years, so she thought that her condition was linked with their exacerbation. Two weeks before her death, she understood everything on her own. She accepted and told me not to feel guilty. Till now I have had tears in my eyes and a scar in my heart. Seeing my mom "in the same boots", I let her doctor tell her everything. She underwent an operation that lasted longer than was planned: stomach resection, several lymph nodes removal, and bowel resection for complicated by stones diverticulitis as an intraoperative finding. After surgery, the biopsy excluded her cancer. One of the happiest moments in medicine, when the initial bad diagnosis is not confirmed! Being with her days and nights, the day before her discharge, I went to sleep at home. While stuck in the traffic, I received a call from her. "Karine, could you come back, please? I feel so bad! I cannot describe what exactly I have, but I do feel bad. I called the nurse, she checked everything and said I am just over worried before upcoming discharge". While I reached her, she developed symmetric breaking pain in her forearms. A non-classical symptom of myocardial infarction! People with diabetes, especially the elderly usually have an atypical presentation. The cardiologist verified the myocardial infarction, and the coronary angiography revealed 99% and 90% occluded coronary arteries. How she survived the long operation! When I left Armenia without knowing that I will stay to live in the United States, both my parents were recovering from their serious illnesses. Now, this pandemic poses a hazard to their well-being and threatens their lives. Unbearable to think I may not see them again. But I do not let the fear take over me. They are alive now; I can talk to them any second and see their smiles on camera. Another reason to be grateful and happy!

July 2020

The calm before the storm

After four months of hard studying, Victor graduates his college within the designated period with the highest grades! To say I am proud of him is to say nothing. I have always believed in him, even though he said he was lazy and did not like studying. We realized that he disliked studying via reading, but listening, practicing, watching were interesting and acceptable for him. Nowadays, there are so many opportunities to learn, plus free time due to the pandemic. One of our credos is "If you are bored, learn something new!". To play a musical instrument, to train a sport or to do a home workout, to learn dancing, cooking, baking, or food carving, to paint, to study a new language, to improve your knowledge as a professional... Everyone has at least one hidden talent, discover it! Whatever you learn, is useful for you and someone else like flowers in your garden delighting others. When we started this journey with Victor, it looked like an adventure, a shared hobby to shorten days during the lockdown. But it turned into a new profession. We are aware that it is just a start, but a good one. There is a necessity to gain practice. One day, hopefully in near future, I and Victor can work together, me as a practicing physician, him - as an allied health professional. I hope Victor's experience can be an example for people self-stereotyped as "lazy" and "far from books".

In general, July is passing relatively still and peacefully at least for me and the people around me. We are used to living with this pandemic. The calm before the storm, unpredicted one!

Just opened my eyes at 6 a.m., I hear someone knocking on my door hard. I and Eddy are alone at home. The noise was so loud that I hardly can hear a man screaming "Open the door". The last evening, we talked with my sisters about the recent protests concerning Black people and the violent clash between Armenians and Azerbaijani in Los Angeles. Hurtful topics for people who are against violence and aggression, who try to create a peaceful and mutually respective environment wherever possible. My sisters asked me whether we are in a safe place and I reassured them. With this background conversation now, I assume that someone escaping from police tries to enter. I see my door almost broken. No time to call 911. Instinctively I am looking for a knife or something heavy to protect me and my son. The shredder is near the door, but I do not reach it. The door opens sharply hitting me. And I see three men uniformed and armed. I still do not understand what is going on, however, feel some relief seeing: at least, not a criminal. While working at the hospital I trained myself to turn off my hearing when someone is screaming and shouting to be able to concentrate on the real problem, the patient's condition, but not the relatives' panic or wildness. With this "professional ability", I could not hear that they were presented themselves and warned if I did not open the door, they would break it. The man who broke the door directs the gun on me and shouts:

- Get out! - like I am a criminal.
- I need to take my son; he is in the crib! – I answer firmly.
- Get out, we will bring him! – he shouts again.

I do not realize how ignoring his command and gun I run to hug Eddy and go outside where I see about eighteen agents of the Federal Bureau of Investigation (FBI) and Homeland Security Investigation (HSI). It is surely not a movie scene, not a joke for a hidden camera, it is real. But why? In a second, I comfort myself "I did nothing wrong, so I am protected". A few minutes later all the neighbors living in the same building gather and the agents start their investigation. When we just moved to this area a few months ago, the first neighbor met welcomed, and assured us, saying "This is a very safe area. I have been living here for about thirty years and I have not seen any criminal". Now we all examine each other with suspicious glances trying to find out the reason for the storm. Eddy, - hungry and with a full diaper, starts babbling with a female officer and neighbors resolving the shock and defusing the tension. Two hours of sitting on the bench, observing their task done professionally, then two weeks of waiting for my iPad to be brought back with all the educational materials for my nurses, and the reason for the storm is revealed - a big bank fraud done by one of the neighbors. I am in disbelief why some people living in the country with rules and rights, million possibilities to grow and to cherish, various social, financial, medical supportive programs, neglect all the benefits and commit a crime, especially now, during these tragical times for the whole world. Trying to win a little, they lose everything… This episode was the analogy happening inside our organism. When some exogenous or endogenous microbes or our cells threaten the whole body, our immune system storms them and cleans up sometimes unintentionally affecting properly working cells. If the protection mechanisms are weakened by other diseases or conditions, microbes win. So, we need to take care of our general health and immune protection every day while we are healthy, and in case if we have already acquired some diseases, to control and manage them as much as it depends on us. Neither our life nor our health is something granted.

This month I find the facts to share with my readers on real COVID-19 cases being much more than registered. The CDC's COVID-19 Response Team reports the outcome of a new study announcing about 10 times more coronavirus infection cases between late March and mid-May, overall, 6-24 times more estimated cases than established. This decreases the real case fatality rate, but again I would like to accentuate that we never know whether we or our beloved ones will be within the smaller percentage or no. Our general duty is to follow all the established preventive measures and to stay safe as much as it depends on us.

These days a lot of people have been following medical news. Acceptable leisure until it does not reach the level of fanaticism. One of the described situations is the debate sparked around vitamin D. The outcome of a large, population-based study about low plasma vitamin D levels as an independent risk factor for coronavirus infection and hospitalization is published. How does a physician understand this information? - To test patients for vitamin D levels (if possible) and if low, administer vitamin D in an individually chosen dose for their overall health. This is not a protective tablet against coronavirus infection! How do nonphysicians (at least many of them) understand this? To run to a pharmacy and buy a lot of vitamin D for the whole family and friends for the upcoming year without understanding real indications or considering side effects and overdose. "Do you have a gift for a relative's birthday?". "Yeah, a big bottle of vitamin D", - humor on this topic. The likewise story regarding vitamin C and zinc. This is a false adaptive mechanism when we seemingly follow medical news and try to become healthier or more protected. We eagerly swallow pills and supplements based on someone's experience or advertisement and falsely comfort ourselves that we care about our health. What about quitting bad habits: smoking, abusing alcohol, using illicit drugs, drinking soda instead of water, eating unhealthy fast food, sitting in front of the TV instead of walking, and so on? Why do we park in front of the entrance instead to walk few feet more especially now when we are not in such a hurry as we were before the pandemic? I do not blame anyone as all of us have at least one poor habit, including me. However, let us not ignore the art of small steps to become healthier and happier.

Unrevealed chain

This month I have my first birthday as a mommy. Victor buys me a gift I have been dreaming of a long time ago and have forgotten for a while. A bicycle! A usual thing for millions, especially in the United States, but I have never ridden a bike. I try to learn on my own but every trial finishes with bruises and a bigger motivation to do it again. Then Victor offers me to take a lesson with a professional instructor. He teaches me just two hints and I learn ridding in less than an hour. An amazing feeling! If you have never tried to do it, follow me as soon as you can.

The backstage I face the previous concerns plus another excessive attitude toward COVID-19 testing. Now, the people who have contacted a person with known or unknown coronavirus status for more than fifteen minutes and within 6 feet (1.8 meters) are afraid and run for testing. According to the latest CDC guidance, these contact persons do not necessarily need to run the test if they are asymptomatic.

- There is nothing bad in being overinsured. Better than to neglect, - people resist.
- It is not forbidden to be tested on your own will, - I answer, - But there is a little chance that the test can catch you at the end of the incubation period or in case if you develop an asymptomatic form of the disease. Nonetheless, let me agree with the CDC's guidance. At first, this kind of over-testing is a burden on laboratory personnel despite your payment. Second, there is a possibility of false-positive and false-negative results. "False positive" signifies that you did not contract the infection, but your test result falsely indicates that you are sick, so you will be forced to follow self-isolation for fourteen days without any symptoms and you will be wrongly counted as an asymptomatic case. A false-negative test result means you are considered healthy and non-infectious for others while being infected.
- Your explanation on possible false results makes sense, doctor, - I receive positive feedback from many of them.

However, I know that some of the responders still do the test uselessly. Educating people, healthcare professionals know that the information cannot be digested at the same required level. Different individuals – different results. But this is an important part of success in medicine. Misunderstanding and poor interaction between a healthcare provider and a patient may ruin all the other parts of the work performed. Even though this job takes me time, my family does not readily accept it, I receive no salary for it, it seems invisible and unrevealed, I know people need it. It is one of the essential parts of effective patient management and infection control. Therefore, I withstand here and continue my self-training and people guiding.

Another war

The fall starts and we start to fall. One of the hardest periods not only during this pandemic but in my life, too. On September 27, early in the morning, I wake up from the loud voice of Victor's phone. It is weird as he never turns the voice on while we are asleep. Something serious happens. I have never seen the sight Victor had at that moment. It expresses mixed feelings; both suddenness and expectation, fear and hope, anger and will to take a gun again. The war between Azerbaijan and Nagorno-Karabakh (Artsakh) resumed. The ceasefire that ended the First Nagorno-Karabakh war (1988-1994) collapsed. The fights have never stopped since then though. We understood that the war may restart any time, but like any other disaster the war never happens "on time". Nagorno-Karabakh, Artsakh, is also Armenia! My mother's uncles and cousins died for their homeland. We have a lot of relatives there, honest people, farmers, military officers, physicians, teachers. I do not want to explain politician games as much as I know, to comment who resumed the war and for what, who is guilty. All these are not in my scope. I just desire to share our story, "the war genealogy". My favorite grandparents were born and lived in Artsakh till their marriage then they moved to Baku, Azerbaijan Soviet Socialist Republic. Their children were born and raised there, including my mom. My grandfather served in Soviet Union Army during World War II and was considered missing in action. My grandmother, a brave woman with immense faith and love, hidden from everyone the news being sure he would come back, and he did. He was found alive among the fallen and saved by Polish women. When he returned home, instead of their little son he found a daughter of the same age he left before going to war. Their little son died suddenly in my grandma's arms when grandpa was at the front and she was pregnant with a girl. A few years later my grandpa died from traumas sequalae received during the war leaving four minor children and a 30-year-old wife a widow. Despite being a beautiful young woman, she was loyal to her husband and did not get married again raising their children with incredible efforts but in love.

I and my sisters are also a generation grown during a war. I was in elementary school and my eldest sister - a high school graduate. We were far from the frontline yet felt all the hardship of the war. Summers were somehow tolerable because the days are long and warm, and daddy was doing his best at the work and in the garden to feed us. We have been in a quite good situation having village products, fruit, and vegetables not only for summer; but also canning, drying, marinating for winter. My uncle, a refugee from Azerbaijan living in the United States had been helping us to his greatest extent possible. So, we could afford to buy some warm clothes and firewood for winter, meat once in several months, and books for education. Winters were intolerable, though people may overcome anything if they have faith and love. The schools were closed during cold months: in Armenia from November till April. First distance education in my life without computers, smartphones, internet. And without electricity! Though we had it but just for an hour per day and every day at different times, sometimes late at night. So, mommy often woke up late at night to cook, wash and bathe us. Bath was via big cup spilling the prewarmed water. We were so lucky to have a 24-hour water supply. In other districts, our relatives had to bring water sometimes from several miles far. For technical usage, they were towing the snow. But what was interesting in these awkward conditions, that I had never seen anyone in our environment with dirty clothes, hair, or bad body odor. We somehow managed to keep hygiene and self-care at their highest level. We were going to school once a week for few minutes to exchange new and done homework. My eldest sister was preparing to enter the faculty of Computer Science at the State University often studying under candle lights. Once she fell asleep while studying and the candle dropped on her book. She was crying when she found out few pages of her handbook burned because the books were more precious than gold then. Then we invented kerosene lamps for safer lessons. Our little stove and some wood gave us a temperature of 55°F (13°C) just in two rooms from four. So, all winter long my parents, three sisters, and I were in the two rooms breathing and living as one organism. As the beds were cold, my mom was singing, and we were dancing to warm up and to be able to jump into the "cold water" that was warmed a bit by daddy for her four daughters one-by-one. After this long journey to his bed, his feet were so cold, that he needed to be warmed. You may think that without electricity we did not watch TV. We did. My dad, an engineer, improvised a small black and white TV with a screen size equal to a modern iPad and bought a small generator giving energy for the 1–2-hour TV session and a small lamp. This was a real harmony I have never met again. Our family, the neighbors' families, overall, about twenty people of different ages and preferences were watching the same TV show or movie for 1-2 hours! By the way, one of our favorites was the soap opera, Santa Barbara. The only fun for all of us among cries from everywhere for their lost beloved ones in the war. Despite these horrendous times, our life was full of so much love, faith, hope, power, friendship, mutual support, empathy hard to find anywhere and anytime else.

My father-in-law volunteered for military service during First Nagorno-Karabakh War. He told to her wife that he was going to a market to buy bread but went straight to the frontline. He came back safe and sound after three months bringing starving soldiers instead of bread. Later he lost almost completely his hearing as a war consequence. My husband served in the armed forces when he turned eighteen during 1993-1994. He was at the hottest battles. He does not like to talk about the hell he saw. Just once he told that one of the last battles before the ceasefire cost them irreplaceable losses. They were 250 people, and just 50 returned. When I asked him how he survived, he answered "God saved my life, otherwise it would be impossible". Few minutes of silence followed, then he added, - "The first victim was my commander who predicted that I would survive. I was bringing ammunition to him, a father of two kids, - and an enemy sniper shot him in the head. I screamed like a wounded beast and my friends removed me from there for few minutes until I recovered from the shock. After the first few deaths either the pain, shock, and all emotions blurred to let you do your functions automatically, or you die because of your fears and excruciating pain in your heart". Victor was announced as a killed in action. Later when the lists were précised it was revealed that his namesake was killed, and Victor was found in the hospital. Now when the war restarted, he is ready to go fighting again but stays because of me and Eddy finding his responsibility against us stronger. After few days of shock due to the worsening news, he manages to detach and goes to work. The Armenian diaspora all over the world help as much as possible, but due to the destroyed system, we understand that there cannot be a positive result for our homeland itself. We just try to reach out to concrete people and somehow weaken their suffering. Girls are sending to unknown soldiers candies with supporting letters, farmers sell their only animals to send money to the frontline, women knitting warm clothes for soldiers, a teenager with no driver license saves his and neighbors family driving them out from the air-raid, a pair gets married at the bombing church, doctors volunteer to the frontline my friends and colleagues among them, children draw and play musical instruments to earn money for the army, a patient with cystic fibrosis who had fully waived from the obligatory military service, volunteer to the army. These are so touching stories that can be continued for hundreds of pages yet are not convenient for this book. We cannot wait to hear about a ceasefire to be announced, however, no harbingers yet.

What do people feel seeing the bombing of their homes, their relatives being killed…? I barely can imagine. The stress reaction after the incident with the FBI stayed for about a month: while the officer was breaking the door, I did not know who was behind it. Those few seconds until I realized who was there were terrible. Once when I was ten-year-old and the war still was going on, we were evacuated late at night due to fire in a military base nearby. We saw, heard, and smell the firearm explosions. Even being a child, I still remember vividly all the feelings of leaving our home without knowing we would come back or no. I also recall our relative from Nagorno-Karabakh who was born and grew up during the 1988-1994 war. A few years later when he visited us and we offered him small dark candies, he became pale, run away, and hid behind the sofa screaming "throw away, it is a gun cartridge". How many broken lives and futile victims, how much aggression, hate, destruction, and hostility…? People, humans, please, stop the wars! No matter who is guilty, who attacks first, what is the aim, where does it happen... Stop it! There are so many other disasters and challenges to overcome: earthquakes, fires, storms, pandemics... In medicine, every disorder has modifiable and unmodifiable risk factors or causes, and we, healthcare workers, do everything to prevent or minimize modifiable ones. And this strategy is more correct, efficient, humanitarian, and cost-effective. War is a modifiable disaster. People who are responsible for it, please, do not allow it to ruin our Organism.

People in Armenia give up wearing masks and keeping social distancing due to war. Deaths from coronavirus and war keep increasing. Hospitals are full of wounded soldiers, the ambulances do not reach urgent patients, like febrile ones. A lot of colleagues who come back from the frontline contracted the coronavirus. In this chaos, my sisters and father also develop COVID-19. I am worried for mom, as well, but it seems her first blood group makes sense. She has a milder form and recovers easily with no complications. Daddy is in worse condition. Before the war, he got an exacerbation of his aplastic anemia and now needs a blood transfusion. But if febrile, it is forbidden to enter the Hematology Center or any other hospital nonspecialized for coronavirus. A vicious circle. I try to organize his care on distance. He does not complain of any symptoms other than fever and headache, but even if he would have just a positive laboratory test with his aplastic anemia, he should receive specialized care. The first ambulance refuses to go to him stating that they are overloaded with soldiers and heavier patients. The second ambulance arrives, checks his temperature and oxygen saturation, and does not take him to the hospital saying that his saturation of 95% is perfect.

This is a warning for all healthcare workers. I have seen this not once when we hurry to sort out people that are not in an emergent situation, but they will be there in a few hours or days and then we hardly can help them. We, medical professionals, have algorithms and guidelines on how to act in these kinds of situations, especially when resources are limited, however, these guidelines are far from being close to ideal. Circumstances that force us to choose between human lives are one of the torturing situations in medicine often leading to burn-out, depression, and even suicides among healthcare workers. During my work at the National AIDS Center of Armenia, I faced with hardest situations and extremely severe or dying patients daily. Being young and not having self-protection mechanisms trained, I reached the burn-out. For me, it was like this: a severe-ill patient admits and you want to run away to a desert island for a few months just not to deal with another challenge, yet you smile and say, "how can I help you today" ... Later I overcame it and one of the tricks was concentrating on saved lives more, than lost ones. One of the reasons I adored and chose infectious diseases as the narrow specialization, that it is "like a surgery but with medications", you can see your dying patient not only overcame the infection, but also recovered completely, transformed, and became younger and happier. Those patients helped me the most then to conquer the burn-out and continue my medical carrier.

I do not give up it even now is far from practical medicine and despite the difficulty to concentrate due to war and chaos in the homeland. In my medical newsletters, I found that two more comorbidities, supported by mostly case series and case reports, have been added to the list of diseases with a significant association of the risk of severe COVID-19 disease: cystic fibrosis and thalassemia. The next day, by a terrible coincidence my student, a young talented pharmacist with thalassemia dies due to COVID-19. And a few days afterward, the coronavirus takes the life of another student who had no diagnosed comorbidity… People go and we even cannot say goodbye…

When will we stop seeing deaths? No one knows. The only things we can do now - to hope, to pray, and to support each other.

October 2020

The lost battle

October is started very actively. There is a lot of medical news that I share and discuss with my friends, students, and colleagues who are eager for updates from me about various aspects of coronavirus infection management.

Remdesivir, one of the antiviral medications that have been evaluated as an effective treatment of COVID-19, is now approved, - and indicated for the treatment of hospitalized adults and children aged 12 years and older with weight 88 pounds (40kg) and more. However, these are just initial data and many concerns are yet to be explored, such as decreased mortality or only improvement of symptoms, hospital stay, etc.

Additional information on positive postinfectious PCR results is received from Italy showing that about 1-in-6 (17%) of people recovered from COVID-19 retest positive for a minimum of two weeks after the disease onset. The presence of two symptoms, sore throat, and rhinitis are more prevalent among them. In other words, people who keep having sore throat and rhinitis, better be assessed for additional PCR tests and be cautious with contacts. What is interestingly found out later is that having the above-mentioned or other symptoms after 2 weeks of recovery, - does not correlate with PCR positivity. It let us suggest that symptoms are not due to ongoing viral replication in many cases. In another small study, the follow-up of the "officially recovered" (two negative test results at least 24 hours apart) patients do not illustrate how positive PCR results correlate with virus viability and contagiousness. Moreover, sore throat and rhinitis were observed in both positive and negative PCR groups. Because of the small sample size of the study, the conclusions were vague. We can resume, if someone with residual symptoms like sore throat and rhinitis, retests positive, for others' sake he is better to be quarantined for a second time until new evidence is revealed.

In October, the outcomes of a German study, not peer-reviewed yet, are published, emphasizing good ventilation technology as the most crucial chain among nonspecific prevention measures lowering the risk of coronavirus spreading at public close-space activities. Wearing face masks and limiting numbers of contacts are accounted as effective preventive practices, as well.

Another challenge appears in October; so-called "twindemic", i.e., the overlap of seasonal influenza outbreaks with coronavirus pandemic. These two viruses share many symptoms and proper laboratory diagnostic is required for adequate management of the patients with co-infection, flu, and COVID-19, as those patients have a higher risk of respiratory compromise than in the presence of either of the two infections. COVID-19 is approximately ten times fatal than the flu. No vaccines against CoV-

SARS-2 are available yet. This points up the role of the flu vaccine during this twindemic, especially in the elderly and people with comorbidities, as well as their family members. I would like to emphasize that a flu shot does not fully guarantee insusceptibility to the flu virus, rather it decreases the chances of catching it, and in case of infection, having a milder form of the disease and lower the risk of being hospitalized. This is particularly important to know, as there can be misunderstanding information spreading among people, like "no sense of being vaccinated. I was vaccinated but contracted flu, it is pointless". And better to receive the flu shot in October as the seasonal increase of flu cases occur in late October till early March. Besides, we must wait for at least two weeks for the flu shot to start working, as well as any other shots.

Having received our flu shots, we go to Las Vegas for few days to take some time out from the overwhelming information coming daily from Armenia. The perfect time for it: the weather is still warm in Las Vegas but not burning and it is not crowded due to the pandemic. I go but my mind is with my daddy. He has been hospitalized a few days ago with a worsened general condition, lung affection, and low oxygen saturation. I am in contact with his attending doctor and hematologist. All decisions concerning his treatment we make together. He has been receiving blood transfusions as indicated based on his hemoglobin level. He is also administered anakinra, an interleukin-1 inhibitor. It is a biologically active substance produced by many cells of our body and regulating inflammatory processes, however, may harm the body if excessive. Its inhibitor is used for severe COVID-19 cases within the framework of clinical trials based on effects observed in small studies.

- Dad, you receive modern treatment and have the best doctor. There is a huge army of admirers waiting for your recovery, - I tell him despite feeling butterflies in my abdomen. I finally hear his voice, at least the voice. He has not been answering for few days because of difficulty breathing, as he explained to my sister. Or maybe he did not want me to see him via the camera in that condition.
- I know, my girl. You are my best doctor. You have already saved my life once…, - I feel some desperation between the lines, - The staff is so attentive and caring, I am surprised and even feeling guilty.
- Why? – I try to precise the reason.
- Karine, there are so many soldiers with serious and multiple injuries lying in the corridor waiting for their turn to be cared for. And me, I am in a private room with the best staff caring for me.
- Dad, you are in a private room to be isolated until your coronavirus test turns negative. Then you will be discharged. Do not concentrate on soldiers now. Try to have a rest, - I tell him bye rapidly trying to hide my tears and intending to call him again soon.

He has been receiving steroids as indicated per guidelines, but they have decreased his low white blood cells fighting against infections even more. We are asked to buy filgrastim, a medication to stimulate his white blood cells to grow and overcome the disease easier. Victor sends money, sisters buy. Everything he needs, we organize emergently. A few days later computerized tomography pictures of lungs and oxygen saturation are improved. We are waiting for PCR test results and prepare him for discharge. But he develops hemoptysis, i.e., coughing up blood. Bronchoscopy shows no problem. He is being prepared for discharge or the transfer to the hematology hospital as soon as his PCR results on coronavirus turn negative. I send him encouraging messages with cute and funny photos of Eddy. That evening I keep trying to reach his phone. Uselessly! No answer again as it was during his first days in the hospital. Eddy is sleeping. Victor offers me a glass of wine and a romantic evening we were dreaming about for the last few weeks.

- I am sorry, Victor, could we postpone it? I feel in my bones that something bad happened with daddy. He is not answering, my sisters and his doctors, as well, - I tell Victor with guiltiness.

- Sure, Karine, - he answers with understanding, - but I guess you are exaggerating. Try to turn off the doctor in your head, please, and have some freshening sleep.

I agree, nevertheless, my sleep is interrupted shortly after. I keep trying to reach someone in Armenia for some news. Short, unnatural group chat conversation with my sisters makes me feel worried more:
- Irina, Bella, Helen, who has some news from dad?
- Everything is ok, he was awake last night because of a cough and now turned off the phone to sleep.
His doctor responds to missed calls from me by the message; "I am at the meeting. I will call you back in an hour". Everything seems explainable, but I write to George, my cousin, who is a friend of daddy's doctor and has arranged my contact with him recently.
- George, I cannot reach daddy for two hours. Sisters said he is sleeping but he never sleeps so long in the morning. His doctor does not answer, as well.
- He talked to me this morning. As I know everything is Ok.
- He talked to you but has not answered my calls? - I persist to know the truth.
- You know, Karine, the uncle developed another stroke, - he writes after a while seemed decades to me.
- What?! What does it mean "another"? He has never had a stroke.
- Oh, sorry, I confused the terms. It was not a stroke, but a heart attack.

- So, he is probably in the intensive care unit, that is why no answer, isn't it? Or is he unconscious?
- No, he is not unconscious…., - a pause follows. George tries to write something. Then I read, - he is not unconscious. He died…! About two hours ago. We could not tell you immediately. Karine, I am so sorry… be strong….

Like the world ruined on my head. I screamed…

I have been dialing him right when he was leaving us. And even was upset of no answer followed. It was a heart attack, probably due to a thrombus. No postmortem examination was performed due to law restrictions concerning coronavirus-positive patients in Armenia. The first and the only unfinished conversation with him was the last one like I tried to escape telling him goodbye.

We are never ready for disasters and losses. We can be educated, trained, having perfect coping mechanisms developed, but the death is never on time. When a happy thing, a newborn, success come into our lives, we take them for granted. When we drive to go to work, shopping, or anywhere else, we are sure we will reach our destination. When we go into the supermarket, we know there will be bread or milk to buy. Going to bed, we do not think that there may be no next morning. I do not encourage being anxious or preoccupied with upcoming possible tragedies. On the opposite, I want to accentuate that whatever we have is a gift to be appreciated, to concentrate more on what we have right now. There should be a balance between preoccupation and readiness to accept bad things as we accept any visible or invisible treasure of our lives. If you lost, if you are heartbroken, or seeing no light at the end of the tunnel, do not blame, do not try to find guilty, do not complain! We cannot bring back our beloved ones and hug them at least for a second, but I believe we will meet them again one day. If you do not believe, please stop, and think. If there is no other life after death and we just disappear, so you will not feel like being "fooled" by your expectation to see your dead beloved ones again. You will not feel anything. But if it is true, why torture yourself with hopelessness while you leave in this world and deprive yourself of hope?! I do believe I will see my father again. And now with this overpowering pain, I feel also immense gratefulness for having him with us, for his perfect fatherhood, for the three additional and full years he was with us after having no chances given by his doctors, for his love, care, and lessons we will keep in our heart while we are alive and even after. I am thankful for my sisters, mother and nephew recovered from the coronavirus, for my husband, for our son. Hugging Eddy every time, I also hug my daddy as Eddy's one-quarter is from the grandpa!

The end of October brings us another grief from Armenia. Victor's cousin died from COVID-19 in the hospital after few days of fight leaving a widow and two minor children. Victor, her sister, and cousins grew together in the same yard as one family. We are a generation that is not used to the word "cousin" rather sister or brother, as my sister Emmy in New York. The death of Victor's brother, almost his peer, is heart-breaking even for Victor who has seen so many deaths in his life. This month is the worst for everyone we have been in contact with lately. Everyone has a loss from either of the wars. Victor finds the power to confess how he was wrong a few months ago when the pandemic had just started. He said, "Karine, all those people, including me, who were saying if the coronavirus is so deadly, why we do not know anyone who died from it, now feel on their skin the pain of the loss, now they know…". I have nothing to say. I hug him being unable to hide my tears.

The sun shines after the rain! And now while we have a chance, we should enjoy every smile of our dearest ones, say sorry if we hurt someone, forgive if we are offended. Enjoy the sky we see, the air we breathe, the warm bath we take, the music we listen to, the tasty tea, coffee, water, or food we drink or eat alone or with someone. Even if we have nothing and no one, we should be thankful for our life, and this day is a chance to be better tomorrow. Remember when we are weak, we are strong. Disasters and tragedies help us see our weaknesses and strengths. What we really can do, becomes evident only when we are in an extremely stressed situation when we fight for our or others' life. We lost the battle but not the war! In this war we are still alive, so we are needed to be here!

Grafting

The war between coronavirus and humans does not tend to come to an end.

The happiest moment this month is Eddy's first birthday. He walks and says few words filling our hearts with joy and light. We organize a small party of ten people not only because of the pandemic, - but due to the narrow list of real relatives who are next to us both in happy and sorrowful times. Neither I nor Victor like big gatherings for family occasions. We have a lot of acquaintances, colleagues whom we are ready to help whenever and however we can, nevertheless, real friends and soulmates count on the fingers of my hand.

Eddy gets his first common cold. The first three days are going as they should be in the one-year-old baby. On the fourth-fifth day usually, it tends to go down, but Eddy is bound to me permanently. He is weak, not eating or drinking despite normal body temperature. He had just one not-heavy diaper in the last twenty-four hours. We are again without Victor being unable to go to a pharmacy. The pediatrician's office again does not answer my calls and messages. I had treated so many pediatric patients with the common cold and other infections, including severe ones. I should be confident, but the physician's parents are also parents. They often need a few simple advice or reassurance, some supportive words. And now I am all alone with my baby with blunted medical information in my head. I and Eddy need some help. I call 911. When I open the door to meet the team, Eddy, attached to me for so long with no positive emotion, starts to smile looking at the blinking lights of the ambulance. The paramedic asks me:

- Ma'am, did you call us for him.
- Yes, - being unable to explain the exact reason.
- For this smiling, happy buddy? Ma'am, sorry but I do not see any indication to take him to the hospital or even a reason why you called us, - he says ready to go. He did not check Eddy's temperature or observe him. He even did not enter. For a second, I try to understand whether I am so fooled by overthinking and exhaustion, - or they do not want to examine him.
- You see, the ambulance staff refused to transport my dad to the hospital stating that his oxygen saturation is perfect. A few days later he died. I see that my son's condition is not so poor but is it normal for a one-year-old baby to have just one partially wet diaper in 24 hours, to drink, or to eat nothing at all for two-three days? If I could reach his doctor, I would not disturb you, - I tell him trying to justify my action.

- I am sorry, ma'am, for your loss. But I see a happy baby who does not need medical attention from our side. Try to contact his pediatrician again. Do you still need us to be here?
- No, sir, thank you for coming. Sorry to bother you from more serious patients, - I add somehow just to be polite.

Eddy recovered within few days but ceased breastfeeding. This was my first experience of dealing with the common cold as a mommy: nothing general with what I have been doing as a physician…

On November 9, an agreement of another ceasefire is signed to terminate all hostilities in the Nagorno-Karabakh area. At first sight, it means no more victims, on the other hand, it announces the unfair loss of a big part of our homeland; refugees; start of another migration wave; poverty; disappointment; thousands of futile killed people fell for our homeland; hopelessness. All my colleagues who have volunteered in the frontline are frustrated and broken as I have never seen them. And not only them but every Armenian living there or abroad who loves that amazing, small, wounded country. The Armenian diaspora is spread all over the world estimated at 8 million with one of the largest populations living in the United States and suffer in the same way despite the distance.

During two years of my stay here I have faced both troubles and favors; highlights and challenges, as equally everywhere less or more expressed. I had periods wishing to go back, but mostly I have been feeling much more confident and complete here. My image of the United States has changed a lot since then. I got married and became a mother here. Even though my husband is Armenian, he is a US citizen living longer in this land than in Armenia. This country accepted and supported us sometimes more than our homeland. When I am asked annoying questions such as "Which country do you love more, Armenia or the United States?", I do not answer. Almost the same meaningless question asked to a kid "Who do you like more, daddy or mommy?". Sometimes, we, diaspora, are being blamed for "leaving our country for one plate of soup". This is so unfair. No one in the world would ever long to leave her or his homeland for no reason. To go abroad for training, higher qualification, exchange, business, education, or tourism, surely. But to quit everything there, to leave everyone and everything we have seen since your birth, and to direct ourselves toward vagueness, does require braveness, faith, and readiness to learn new things almost daily. Every emigrant has his or her own story and reason. Mine is seemingly simple. Every person has responsibilities toward parents, homeland, spouse, children, and society. The latter we realize via our job, profession, talents, and abilities. When there is neither balance between these responsibilities, functions, realization, and feedback, nor perspective, it is a way to a foreign country. During the hardest period in Armenia 1988-1994 my parents, both skilled engineers, received multiple invitations from various countries, but they stayed despite indescribable difficulties because they were hopeful that it was just a period to be resolved and overcame. As for me, I stopped feeling progressing as a professional and seeing any perspective. Most of the time I knew the clues and the steps for my patients' treatment and wellbeing but was in chains. I was also fed up with working days and nights, combining practical and academic jobs that I adored but receiving a miserable salary, being unable to buy even medications for my parents or take them for a deserved trip; trying to develop the healthcare system, - but with no support. In my opinion, it is equal to the inheritance of great property but unable to use it. My crucial decision was followed by gigantic work done to suit all the requirements for foreign medical professionals in the United States. Unfortunately, many foreign medical graduates do not manage to overcome these obstacles and unwillingly become taxi drivers, servants, housemaids, nannies, or maximum, paramedics and nurses. They are being lost as physicians both for their country and the United States. I still need to pass medical residency to receive a physician license, but my theoretical knowledge improved much more here with all opportunities to train, study online, continue postgraduate education. As I have already told you, I came to the United States for the USMLE step 2 cs. It is an examination when a medical student or physician needs to evaluate twelve "patients", i.e., actors pretending patients, make initial diagnoses, consult them, administer proper analysis, and write down the results of encounters. Me, who has taught foreign medical students in Armenia for eight years, was considered good in English. When I entered the room where other examinees, native Americans, were waiting to start the exam, I wanted to run away. I understood just 50-60% of their conversation. The worker who was responsible for the proper exam course, a Black man who I would not forget, noticed I was embarrassed. He supported me with a sincere smile and said, "Do not worry, your patients are waiting for you, doctor". This boosted my self-confidence. I hardly could understand some of the patients due to the difference between British and American accents. For a second, I intended to leave the exam. But then I thought "What do I lose if stay and try?". The last USMLE, step 3, is a two-day exam with eight and nine-hour duration and is generally passed by medical residents before they can get their license. I passed it without residency or local training, sitting at home, and studying on my own. I went for the exam being seven-month pregnant with a high-risk pregnancy. My hands were so swollen that the detector could not recognize my fingerprints, then we arrange somehow the issue. I passed all of the USMLEs with average or good scores and from the first attempt. A few sentences to describe that no one leaves the homeland for "one plate of soup" and the way to success abroad is not that easy seemed from far.

A new life in a new country, even in such a developed and powered one as the United States, I would describe it like transplantation of a vital organ, such as the heart, lungs, kidneys, liver, that stopped functioning properly. With a compatible donor organ, ill people receive a second chance. They usually become happier and more thankful than when they were healthy. However, they will never be the same. For the rest of the life, they will need to take "strong" medications and precautions for the transplanted organ not to be rejected.

The sun shines and the rain wets all of us. No matter where we live, but how we live matters. And I am not about a higher salary or more comfort. I am about happiness, gratefulness, self-realization, effectiveness, and love. It is naively said that beauty will save the world. Beauty is a matter of taste! It is Love that will save the world!

December 2020

The end and the new beginning

I and Eddy enjoy Christmas lights and decorations. We made our Christmas tree on the wall and decorated it together. Yes, this Christmas is going to be unforgettable in both negative and positive meanings. We have still isolated at least physically; no family gathering, no shopping, no gifts. But so many people lack family, home, health, money, even hope. Me, I am blessed to have family, relatives, and friends physically close or far, the roof over my head, the ability to move, to talk, to creatc, and to love. A candle loses nothing by lighting other candles. So, I invented a way to do small kind things to strangers. But I will keep it in secret.

I finished drafting our article about COVID-19 influence on operated patients, the results of a cohort study that we have performed with my friend John from February 1 till October 31. It is published as a preprint, not peer-reviewed yet. Even if it stays in this stage, I am satisfied with the first scientific work we have performed being on the other sides of the globe, having received the results, that would be important at least for few people. Additionally, we have gained huge experience for further works.

My online consultations and explanations go on without ceasing. Same concerns globally with another wave of hopelessness and panic. In the United States, there are already more than 16 million people infected and about 300 000 deaths due to coronavirus. We wait impatiently for the vaccines to be released for population use. And here it is! On December 14, the happy news is announced: the first coronavirus shot is injected outside trials in New York. The brave woman who received the first vaccine is the critical care nurse who lost about 30 patients during this pandemic. It seems to be the start to end the pandemic, though another year minimum will be required to win the war. I feel that a lot of positive changes in the world will occur in the new year, as well as, that a new member of our family will be welcomed soon.

January 2021

A new life in the New Year

New Year 2021 is not like others… When the pandemic started, many people said that the world would never be the same again afterward. I do not know what exactly they meant, but I suggest that only a few of us will be transformed into our best. During and shortly after each catastrophe the world is seemingly changed but we tend to forget both bad and good things later. This is probably good unless we forget the details, the emotions, but keep the lessons learned. A child does not remember all the falls and cries while learning to walk but fixes the result and keeps walking. We will forget a lot of things, but please, accept both hard or delighted days as a gift, a new chance to live a better and fuller life, to support, help and love each other more!

On January second, we already have the facts of my second pregnancy. A new human is developing to come into our world!

This month the coronavirus among millions also affects our neighbors, the nurses who I have been training for RN exam, Victor's eldest cousin, and his wife. Though it can be scary for me and my few-week pregnancy, I am not afraid. I limit contacts as much as possible and I keep praying for all known and unknown patients to recover. The Santa we hang on the window will continue to shine and smile until our severely ill dear friends, the neighbor, and Victor's cousin, will be discharged from the hospital safe and sound.

February 2021

Not the same virus?

One of my hobbies is studying foreign languages. English is one of my favorites, but there is an expression I do not accept; "How old are you?". Why old? Couldn't we ask instead "How young are you?". On the other hand, we are getting older since our first day of life. And we know that despite the progress level we will never overcome death. Yet the age is a relative term. There are people 65+ doing much more than others in their youth, and there are people aged 25, wasting their energy for nothing. Sadly, being elderly is one of the risk factors for severe forms of COVID-19. Our neighbor, a 65-year-old man with several comorbidities, a working and creating person who can construct a building with his own hands, has been in the hospital for about a month. Doctors have fought for his life. The Santa's lights have been on every evening waiting for him… until February 5. As a physician dealing with life-threatening conditions, I saw many incredible recoveries, better to say miracles. This time the miracle did not happen. His wife and my mother said the same words that would sound in my ears forever "If I knew that my half would leave me so early, we would spend more time together. We have never had time for ourselves. The time spent with our dearest ones, the actions showing love and respect, the precious memories are all we can carry with us after death".

COVID-19 associated deaths are so excessive that people should wait for weeks to bury their relatives, a supplementary reason to grief harder and longer…

Victor's cousin, whose younger brother died of coronavirus infection in October, has been in severe condition with comorbidities and poor prognosis, however, is now discharged for further recovery at home. He said: "I felt on my skin why my brother was not responding to our calls while in the hospital and what he was feeling before death". This is another miracle, another victory!

The new challenge follows the resolved ones. Now Eddy becomes febrile till 104°F (40°C) with some catarrhal and gastrointestinal symptoms. He cries inconsolably. Again, we are together with him without Victor. The grandparents want to come to help us, but I cannot exclude coronavirus, so I force them to stay at home. They came and left some food and medications behind the closed door and went. I cannot reach the pediatrician's office again. I am several weeks pregnant. I do not know what may happen to us. Eddy and I are vaccinated against flu, the fact giving me some relief (a vaccinated person with flu would probably have less fever) and narrowing his possible diagnosis. It can be either COVID-19, - or human herpesvirus 6 causing the disease named sudden exanthema. On the 4th day, he keeps being febrile despite antipyretics already given in full daily dose. I again call 911. This time the staff is very attentive and professional. They advise me to look for dynamics and give some reassurance that I needed the most. The next day, Eddy's temperature decreases, - and a rash develops on his skin, a course that makes me relax. It is characteristic of the sudden exanthema, a sickness that is almost always observed in little kids.

I keep staying at the backline as a reserve officer. The most frequent question now concerns vaccines. Two doses of Pfizer and Moderna vaccines are necessary to develop adequate immunity against coronavirus within 3 and 4 weeks after the first dose, accordingly, but not late than 6 weeks. If someone for some reason, for example, travel, cannot wait, four days earlier are allowed for the second dose. The vaccines are effective against several new variants, however, there is a possibility of some strains' "escape" the vaccines. How long it will take to develop effective herd immunity; will the mutant strains of the virus escape the vaccine; will the combination of available vaccines increase its effectiveness; how can we protect children? – all these questions are waiting for the answers.

More questions than answers

The nurse who had two fails before I have trained her, - passes the RN exam, - and receives a desired job invitation. I am proud and happy for her. This was a real battle with circumstances: three minor children of different ages stuck at home with no school or kindergarten. She got coronavirus infection a month before her exam, tried to postpone uselessly, but then recovered and did it! We hardly have been managing to meet for new topics and unclear questions once per ten days trying to concentrate while our husbands were taking care of our kids. The rest was done via phone while cooking, cleaning, and doing other chores. Eddy, as a little healthcare professional, has been copying me drawing on papers, - and indicating on medical images. This was an interesting, exciting, and funny period. I am happy to be a motivation for her and have a part in her success.

This month is quite hard for me due to activated antiscientific waves. The law of balance and harmony allows opposite processes exist together: kindness and evil, love and hate, birth and death, health and sickness, science and antiscience. But during this pandemic, antiscientific directions are dominating over the scientific ones. People, do you know that antiscience does kill! Working with HIV dissidents was one of the hardest aspects of my profession, - when people living with HIV refuse not only essential treatment, - but also the existence of the virus and the disease. Peer consultation played a positive role on some percentage of HIV dissidents in our practice, yet not on everyone. When people address to doctors in the late stages of the disease or with a disease that we still cannot treat, it is real sorrow. But losing patients just because their mind tells them lies is much more pitiful, unfair, and unacceptable. During this pandemic, I have been hearing so many antiscientific thoughts wondering where they are coming from. Five months after my dad's death I still receive questions from my sisters and relatives "what if we would do this or that?", questions that have no sense and will change nothing, however, I patiently answer them with available facts. This time the conversation started like this:

- Many people who lost their dears at the hospital report sudden death after evident improvement, as it happened with your daddy. We think that there is a universal program using medical institutions to kill people… That is why we do not let anyone else go to the hospital.

I am about to explode, but remembering my father's patience, forgiveness, and kind smile, I calm down and explain:

- Cases described as "sudden" death in COVID-19 are due to thromboembolic complications into vital organs: heart, brain, lungs, that happens at later stages of the disease when the processes in most affected organs, the lungs, regress, and the general condition is improved. Nothing mysterious or suspicious, - I say not persuading all but at least some of them.

I will not tell everything linked with this topic, as I find too much attention and real facts pose more opposition to growth. However, I will be like water that wears away a stone!

Some concerns around COVID-19 vaccines are being cleared, but the new ones are being added. For effective herd immunity that will let us put coronavirus infection in the range of "a usual seasonal infection", 70-80% of the population is required to be immunized. As vaccines are still not accepted for use in children, only around 75% of the United States population is eligible to be immunized. Excluding people who will refuse the vaccination, we receive about 71-72%. If the mutant B.1.351 or some other variant resistant toward our vaccines dominates, then vaccine-derived immunity is estimated to reach just about 40%. Postinfectious immunity is not able to cover up the gap, as only 19% of the United States habitats have been infected. At least some of them also will need to boost their immunity with vaccination, if not everyone. Masks and social distancing will be required for the upcoming winter 2021-2022, but predictively the level of compliance will be lower due to public tiredness. These are just thoughts based on experts' opinions, predictions, and literature data. We still scramble the mountain and one day will reach the peak, but what exactly we are going to face and how long it is going to take us, no one knows for sure yet.

April 2021

To be or not to be vaccinated?

Eddy got another common cold. This time I do not escape the virus and my condition is worse than his. And again, as already a family tradition, Victor is out of the city on a mission trip. We love him so much that gets sick when he is not home to protect him. Every situation can be accepted with humor and positivity, and this one, too. We cannot reach our doctors and stay at home isolated with "common cold" diagnosed by myself. Happily, after four quite hard days of the illness, we start to recover with no consequences on my pregnancy.

It has been more than a year since the pandemic begins. Long enough to talk about post coronavirus sequelae. A study from Sweden reports that approximately 80% of hospitalized patients with COVID-19 have persistent symptoms at least eight months after the disease onset. The most prevalent symptoms described are loss of smell or taste, fatigue, and shortness of breath. Interestingly the permanent symptoms are common even in people with mild forms of COVID-19 and derange their social, personal, and professional life, including that of healthcare professionals. A study about increased mortality in the United States within March-July 2020 period makes us think even more. The excessive deaths accounted for 20%, 72.4% of which were to COVID-19. The rest 27.6% were due to non-COVID-19 causes, including heart disease, Alzheimer's disease (type of dementia), diabetes. The information being received during the pandemic, - indicates that we are still children in understanding the whole impact of coronavirus on the world. If we leave economic, financial, and other non-medical consequences to be discussed by professionals in corresponding fields, we will still see enormous problems accompanying the pandemic that will last long after. How long can post-COVID syndrome last, how does it manifest, how strong does it affect our daily life? What kind of coronavirus vaccine-associated late sequelae will we observe? How will we deal with collateral damage, such as lower level of other vaccinations, that may lead to outbreaks when a community comes back its previous activity; decreased awareness concerning noninfectious disease screening and prevention, for example, malignancies, cardiovascular diseases, diabetes, obesity, dementia, psychiatric and psychological problems; disturbance in addictions' treatment? This list is quite long and overwhelming. Another study started several years before this pandemic evaluated the suicide risk in patients treated in intensive care units (ICU) versus non-ICU patients. The results were published recently and indicated higher risk in the first group. Imagine, how many people have survived COVID-19 being treated in the ICUs and how careful we need to be with them. Saying "these people have a higher risk for this and that" can seem pointless or exaggerated, but we need to take precautions and be more attentive to risk group people. It is similarly crucial as driving wiser and slower in poor weather conditions.

In a British journal, another interesting study results are published. It turned out that more exercise was linked to a lower chance of severe COVID-19. Compared with individuals who exercised at least 150 minutes weekly, inactive patients had 2.3 times higher chances to be hospitalized, 1.7 times – to be admitted to an intensive care unit, and about 1.5 times more likely to have lethal outcomes. Again possibilities, likelihood… A lot of people procrastinate in starting a new healthier life. Most of them argue that there are so many diseases, so many factors, poor genetics, and so on, that "my efforts of quitting a bad habit are wiped out by them, so no sense to torture myself". How long are we going to lie on ourselves with these kinds of excuses? We can do whatever depends on us and let the rest go as it will. Better safe than sorry! I want to accentuate that regular physical activity is one of the nonpharmacological effective methods in the management of four "famous" risky comorbidities for severe forms of coronavirus infection - cardiovascular disease, obesity, hypertension, and diabetes. I have been slightly or moderately overweight in my life, for example during stressful examination periods and sleepless nights at the hospital, or while breastfeeding. I am a very compliant, strong-willed, and perseverant person, however, even for me starting to fight against the problem was not easy. On the other hand, it is so pleasant to see the results, even the minuscule ones, to feel healthier and have more energy day by day. People, your mood raises with movements, many problems that were preventing you from the lifestyle changes just disappear, you start to like your job or find one, your relationship with others ameliorates, and so on and so on. Many years ago, I learned to compare myself just with one person, me – who I was yesterday and who I can be tomorrow. What can I do today? So, please, dear all, become your hero today, do one unpleasant healthy thing, and do not do one pleasant unhealthy thing today! Then repeat it day by day. One day you will see your health and whole life improved.

This month debates around serious adverse effects of vaccines in various countries, including the United States, such as thromboembolic complications, explode. Unfortunately, rare but severe and life-threatening outcomes are observed after all available vaccines. Nonetheless, the percentage is low, - and compared with possible harms due to the disease itself, the vaccination benefits heavily overweigh the risks. For some vaccines, for example, AstraZeneca's production, risk-benefit outweighing among people younger than 30-year-old is still questionable. I do not intend to criticize any of the vaccines or to add up to people's concerns, but when I am being asked, I share the objective medical information received from all over the world. The observations and updates are continuous, so we need to be more patient and not spread panic. The available coronavirus vaccines are effective despite many other questions that will be elicited in near future.

The scent of victory versus false comfort

This month many questions come regarding coronavirus transmission predominantly via aerosols; social distancing; and treatment with monoclonal antibodies. The information on these topics is being updated quite rapidly.

- Doctor Karine, I have read that social distancing is useless as the main way of coronavirus transmission is via small particles that may spread further than 6 feet (1.8 meters).
- As it was assumed earlier, aerosols appeared to be the main transmission mode of SARS-CoV2, hence social distancing of 6 feet becomes questionable, particularly for indoor spaces with inadequate ventilation. Till now many data proving the effectiveness of adequate indoor ventilation along with social distancing and proper mask-wearing to slow down the transmission rates. The question yet to be answered is about the distance: how far it should be 2 feet, 6 feet, or 20 feet?
- Do the masks protect us from these aerosols?
- As it was already told not once, usual masks cannot completely prevent the aerosols to move through them, yet with other preventive measures compliant mask-wearing decreases the virus spread speed. It makes sense.
- What to expect then?
- Upcoming weeks we will receive the order about less tight restriction concerning social distancing and masks wearing at least outdoor, mostly attributable to increasing levels of vaccination.
- Is it true that monoclonal antibodies are effective for COVID-19 treatment? Patients just need to reach places where it is given.
- This is a bit exaggerated conclusion. Despite some differences between monoclonal antibodies (mAbs) choice, dose, and indications in guidelines of reputable organizations, all of them recommend using mAbs for outpatient individuals with mild-to-moderate COVID-19 who are at high risk for clinical progression. So, the mAbs are not a panacea.
- These groups are the same risk groups for severe disease?
- Almost. Eligible for mAb treatment patients are individuals aged 65 and higher with no additional requirements, or younger people with one comorbidity.
- Such as Alzheimer's disease, psoriasis, rheumatic diseases along with common ones?
- Well, here is the actual list:

- people aged 55-year or more with either one: cardiovascular disease; hypertension; chronic obstructive pulmonary disease, or another chronic respiratory disease.
- children aged 12 or higher with either of these conditions: body mass index (BMI) higher than 35 kg/m^2; chronic kidney disease; diabetes; immunosuppressive disease or current immunosuppressive therapy.
- Individuals within 12-17-year age range with one of the following: BMI higher than 85th percentile; congenital or acquired heart disease; severe asthma or another chronic respiratory disease; neurodevelopmental disorders; sickle cell disease; conditions requiring technological support such as special tubes, respiratory support, etc.

- Wow, this is impressive. It indicates a huge work done in this field.
- Yes. And fresh information continues to be published.
- If someone is treated with antibodies, no need for vaccination, right?
- No, false. Monoclonal antibodies or convalescent plasma provide the organism with protection developed outside of the body. Being proteins, they are destroyed in our organism within a few weeks or months. Meanwhile, vaccines stimulate our immune defense against the virus or other germs. People who recovered from coronavirus infection should receive the vaccine to boost their immunity, however, those who have been treated with monoclonal antibodies or convalescent plasma, - should postpone the vaccination for 90 days after the above-mentioned treatment not to interfere with the vaccine.
- When is one considered fully vaccinated?
- After seven days of the second dose.
- There is an opinion that vaccinated people may acquire COVID-19, - but have no symptoms, meaning missed cases promoting virus transmission.
- For every controllable infection (i.e., one that we have an effective vaccine against it), vaccinated people may become asymptomatic carriers and be contagious. However, the number of them is much lower than imagined. Regarding coronavirus, the vaccination is associated with a notably lower incidence of both symptomatic and asymptomatic cases versus non-vaccination as shown, for instance, in a study that included almost seven thousand healthcare workers in Tel Aviv, Israel.

Everyone waits impatiently for the day when all the questions will be resolved and we can announce our victory, however, not everyone readily goes to receive the vaccine. We forget what we have faced within the first year of the pandemic. Being afraid of vaccination and ignoring the risk from the disease itself is pseudo protection, false comfort. "Let others risk, and I will collect the harvest" principle has never worked.

The healthcare professionals receiving first shots had concerns, too, yet the desire to end up the hell they dealt with was stronger. We are the chains within the same organism. The big day depends on each of us!

June 2021

One more sunrise

On June 15, 2021, California terminates Stay Home Order and reopens the economy. Many restrictions, such as physical distancing, capacity limits on businesses, end up. Still ongoing pandemic checks our lessons learned to let us transfer to the next level or to be retested again and again? Do you know that not only pathologic microorganisms are being transmitted among humans, but good and healthy ones, too? Similarly, not only negativity is "infectious" but also courage, peace, kindness, love, support, respect, creativity, and all other positive things. We have reached this point due to heroes working not only at hospitals, outpatient offices, laboratories, but everywhere, as every vaccinated person is a hero. He or she did whatever should be done for his own and everyone's sake.

Meanwhile, many people are rather at the stage of "collecting information" than real steps to the general win.

- Does the vaccination let us leave our masks?
- Not exactly. They are still required to be worn in public indoor places, such as schools, daycares, hospitals, shelters, public transport, even if fully vaccinated.
- What is the difference then? Not too much to be glad of?
- In fact, this is a big move forward mostly due to the successful vaccination campaign to be continued.
- So many scary cases are linked with vaccines, even some countries ban vaccination.
- This is a normal course for every new vaccine or medication. As many people receive it, more mild or severe side effects will be observed in the population. As a result, the vaccine can be revoked, suspended, or corrected.

Many blame and concerns come from the countries where AstraZeneca's vaccine is the one or the only available option. I am not a vaccination expert. I know that thromboembolic complications, which are characteristic of coronavirus infection itself, have been described following vaccination, particularly (but not only) AstraZeneca's. Denmark is the first country that stopped using AstraZeneca's COVID-19 vaccine since April 2021. At the beginning of April, 169 cases of brain blood clots named cerebral venous sinus thrombosis, were reported after 34 million doses in Europe. A rare, but life-threatening complication which absolute numbers will increase with more people receiving it. Interestingly, the clot may develop within two months after vaccination, thus if postvaccination control is not tight, the numbers can be inaccurate and unreliable. Many countries initially suspended vaccination with AstraZeneca's vaccine, then have weighed the risk-benefit ratio and have resumed it with restrictions linked with age recommending it mostly to individuals older than 50, in some countries – 30, in others – 60. Nevertheless, this June there are initial data published that AstraZeneca's and Pfizer-BioNTech's vaccines are effective against mutant variants and its versions B.1.617.1 and B.1.617.2. Evidently, as with any preventive or curative intervention, we need to follow the principle "Not harm" considering pros and cons, such as the age of people, comorbidities and risk of severe COVID-19, the countries budget, and ability to monitor for side effects in long-term, the mutant variant distribution, availability of alternatives, and so on. Still, hundreds of deaths occur due to coronavirus daily in the U.S., nearly all are in unvaccinated people. Many other countries with low vaccination levels and strategies have worse situations. The overall cases including lethal ones tend to decrease all over the world, but it is still early to talk about the final battle. The vaccination level of less than fifty percent in the United States along with business opening, many canceled restrictions, and activated travels cannot exclude the possibility of a rapid increase of COVID-19 cases with all consequences. Thus, our awareness and responsibilities as humans and professionals should not wane.

The objective and detailed explanation is accepted enough effectively, though I need not only to refresh my knowledge daily, - but also to repeat and repeat the same information that I do readily. The most interesting updates this month are the new risk factors for severe COVID-19 identified, such as poor sleep habits. Moreover, some atypical symptoms, for example, some dermatological manifestations, tend to be removed from the possible clinical picture of the coronavirus infection.

The second year of the pandemic will let us discover, correct, and accomplish a lot of things. The performance is about to end though at a snail's pace. I wish everyone patience, care, peace, and courage until we will stand and applaud.

I am scheduled for vaccination on my seventh month of pregnancy. I learned driving and, in a few days, I have a driving test. My documents are ready to apply for the United States internal medicine residency programs in September. Where does my boat will sail to? I do believe it will be the best place for me and my family.

***

These are eighteen months of the pandemic described by an infectious disease physician backstage, a mother of the family, a daughter, a wife, a human being, one cell in the milliard-cell organism. Each month was like a year for everyone. So, we are legally adults now, hence, we can vote, we can join the military, we can have some freedom, and as an adult, be more responsible, experienced, and aware!

The sun rises again and is even brighter. Who knows how long and how warm the sun will shine? Now it is time to use our solar batteries do our best!

References

1. *JAMA: The Journal of the American Medical Association.* Issues January 2020 – June 2021.
   https://jamanetwork.com/journals/jama.

2. Medscape Infectious Diseases. (January 2020 – June 2021). Updates. News and Perspectives. CME and Education.
   https://www.medscape.com/infectiousdiseases

3. DKBMed Continuing Medical Education for Health Care Providers. (2020, January 1- 2021, June 31). Updates on COVID-19 Treatment. Monoclonal Antibodies 101. COVID-19 in the Pipeline Therapeutics. COVID-19 Patient Case Study Challenge.
   https://dkbmed.com/

4. Centers for Disease Control and Prevention. (2020, January 1- 2021, June 31). Data and Cases: COVID-19.
   https://covid.cdc.gov/covid-data-tracker/#datatracker-home

5. World Health Organization. (2020, January 1- 2021, June 31). Reports and Guidelines: COVID-19.
   https://www.who.int/emergencies/diseases/novel-coronavirus-2019

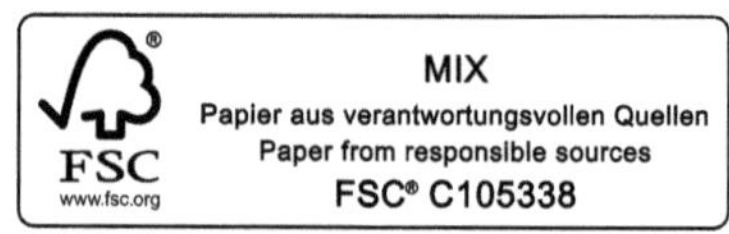

Printed by Books on Demand GmbH, Norderstedt / Germany